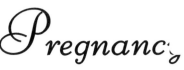

Pregnancy Bedrest

A Journey of Love

A Guide to Managing the Physical,
Emotional, and Spiritual Struggles of a Medically
Challenged Pregnancy

Wanda Hale, MAMFT

Two-Time Bedrest Patient and Mental Health Provider

Forewords by:
Steven M. Beverly, M.D., OB-GYN
Pamela K. Schubarth, RPT

LCI
PRESS

ఴఴఴఴఴఴఴఴ

Pregnancy Bedrest: A Journey of Love
Published by L&C Inspirations, LLC Press
P.O. Box 50768 Bowling Green, KY 42102-3968

Visit our website at
www.LandCinspirations.com
www.PregnancyBedrestEssentials.com

Printed in the United States of America

Hale, Wanda
Pregnancy Bedrest: A Journey of Love/ Wanda Hale, MAMFT; forewords
by Steven M. Beverly, M.D., OB-GYN, and Pamela K. Schubarth, RPT

ISBN 0-9774796-0-9

Contents

ৰ্কীৰ্কীৰ্কীৰ্কীৰ্কীৰ্কীৰ্কীৰ্কীৰ্কীৰ্কী

Publisher's Note of Warning

Forewords

Mrs. Hale's outlook on bedrest treatment in pregnancy is a very practical explanation. Her view, as detailed in her book, describes very practical issues that the mother-to-be may be facing. Her experience with bedrest allows her to offer helpful tips on dealing with this stressful time. She explains the different aspects of bedrest in a way that women can understand, without confusing them with medical terms or jargon. This book will be very helpful to the expectant mother who is nervous about the conditions surrounding, not only her pregnancy, but bedrest treatment as well.

Steven M. Beverly, M.D., OB-GYN

When Wanda told me she was going to write a book on pregnancy bedrest – I thought it was a wonderful idea and a much needed and valuable resource. She has first hand experience with pregnancy bedrest – twice to be exact, and truly wants to help make the pregnancy bedrest journey less stressful for all women who undertake this enormous task. In addition to her own personal experiences with pregnancy bedrest, she has provided care to individuals suffering from emotional struggles during a life crisis through her years as a mental health therapist. Therefore, she has a wealth of knowledge to share. She has written this book to address the woman as a whole – physically, emotionally, and spiritually. In her writing, she provides education on the medical aspects of pregnancy bedrest, physical therapy exercises for the patient on bedrest, coping strategies for the emotional challenges a woman and her family might possibly struggle with during the bedrest journey, and encouragement to look inside oneself and find strength when life situations are not ideal. Her goal is to help women do more than just survive from day to day. She encourages women to accept their life situation and allow growth and knowledge to come from the experience, thereby, embarking on the pregnancy bedrest journey with hope rather than despair. She encourages the woman experiencing a medically challenged pregnancy to turn her obstacles into opportunities.

Having been a physical therapist for twenty years, I have cared for many patients experiencing bedrest for various medical conditions, and I have observed first hand how quickly the human body can experience muscle weakening and cardiovascular de-conditioning when activity levels are decreased drastically. I, personally, feel that a thorough, safe physical therapy program approved by the patients OB-GYN can be very beneficial for the woman experiencing pregnancy bedrest. Physical therapy exercises will aid in maintaining muscle strength and reducing muscle pain, stiffness, and strain, providing sensory input to the body which is significantly decreased during prolonged periods of inactivity and bedrest, as well as preventing circulatory problems. In addition to the physical benefits of exercise, the woman can benefit emotionally as well. After observing patients who have been in bed for extended periods of time, it is obvious the toll that inactivity takes on the person as a whole and not just physically. It is important to emphasize the need for a doctor's approval before beginning any exercises when dealing with a high risk pregnancy, as every woman's condition is unique to her. What might appear safe may actually bring harm to an already threatened pregnancy. So, get a doctors approval first! And, as Wanda has noted in *Pregnancy Bedrest: A Journey of Love*, the body is resilient. After the baby is born, begin re-building physical strength and condition.

Pregnancy Bedrest: A Journey of Love is an excellent resource for the woman and her family faced with the challenges of pregnancy bedrest. Pregnancy should be a time of joy and celebration. If pregnancy bedrest has stolen your joy, reclaim it with this book!

Pamela K. Schubarth, RPT

Acknowledgements

ᘒᘒᘒᘒᘒᘒᘒᘒᘒᘒ

To my husband, Jon, a man of much character, commitment, sacrifice, and who has great love for his family. Where my life would be if you were not in it is a corner of the world to which I hope never to venture. Our family is wonderful, and you play a very significant role in that gift. Thank you for all you have done and will do as we travel the journey of marriage and parenting together. You are not only my partner, but my best friend as well.

To my in-laws, Shirley and Earl, you were knights in shining armor when I needed you most. Thank you for acknowledging the gift of life and for understanding how that gift of life would affect all of our lives. You are wonderful people, parents, and grandparents. Forever, I will be grateful for your sacrifices for our family.

To my children, Lydia and Caleb, an unknown author once wrote, *A baby is a kiss from heaven blown from the hand of God.* You are my kisses from heaven. When I look into your young eyes I see the goodness God created in humans. Your innocence, sweetness, and love have helped me become the person I am and want to be. Thank you for the love, healing, and growth you have brought into my life. I love you with all my being!

To my other family and friends, thank you for supporting me during this venture. Your insights and suggestions have helped to make this book possible. I will forever be blessed for having you as a part of my life.

To Sue Wilson, your kindness in reviewing and editing my book is greatly appreciated.

Introduction

If you are reading this book, you are likely in the same situation as other women – experiencing pregnancy bedrest. My goal in writing this book and developing the Pregnancy Bedrest Essentials set is to help women with the physical, emotional, and spiritual struggles that become a daily part of the bedrest journey. While the ultimate goal is to do everything to help your baby survive and be healthy, it's also important to remember the mother's health and sanity in this process. While this book in no way guarantees the perfect outcome to pregnancy bedrest, I hope it will provide a sense of peace, hope, and comfort as you travel this journey.

In Chapter One, *Author's Pregnancy Bedrest Memoir*, I have taken the opportunity to share my own personal experiences with pregnancy bedrest and how the journey challenged me to look inside myself and move from simply surviving from day to day to living and growing. I share the struggles, as well as the good times. I hope to remind the reader that out of a challenge comes personal growth.

Chapter Two educates the expectant mother to common *Medical Reasons for Pregnancy Bedrest*, as well as to the *Different Types of Pregnancy Bedrest*. Additionally, a list of *Questions for Your Doctor* is provided to help in understanding the exact limitations of the pregnancy bedrest prescription.

Tips for Managing and Coping with Pregnancy Bedrest is presented in Chapter Three. The focus of this chapter is to provide the expectant mother with information on how to make her resting place as comfortable as possible by listing all of the items she might need during her bedrest journey, and by giving suggestions for coping during this challenging time.

Taking care of oneself during a crisis can be hard enough, and having the responsibility of caring for others, especially children, can make life even more stressful. The goal in Chapter Four is to provide education, suggestions, and encouragement to the expectant mother who will be *Parenting Young Children While on Bedrest*.

Chapter Five details the *Common Emotions Experienced* by a woman facing a lengthy bedrest period, along with *Suggestions for Emotional Relief*. Having one's life changed in what feels like an instant can bring with it anxiety, grief, anger, fear, and depression, as well as other emotions. Learning to acknowledge, process, and manage these emotions is beneficial for the expectant mother's physical and emotional wellbeing.

Chapter Six educates the expectant mother to the *Benefits of Relaxation, Relaxation Techniques*, and *Positive Thinking*. The goal in this chapter is to help the bedrest patient explore relaxation and understand how it can bring positive aspects to life, while calming the body and mind from the stress and fear brought about by a medically challenged pregnancy. Learning to relax is an art and a gift and something worth exploring.

Lying in bed for weeks and months takes its toll on the body. As a result of the reduction in physical activity, the expectant mother's body becomes fatigued, tense, and painful. Chapter Seven provides *Exercises for Pregnancy Bedrest* and tips for *Maintaining Energy and Decreasing Muscle Strain* for the bedrest mother. Before performing any exercise listed in this book or elsewhere, get your OB/GYN's approval. Each woman's pregnancy is different, and what might work for one woman may not work for another.

When faced with a crisis, people often ponder the deeper meaning of life and the significance the crisis brings to their spiritual functioning. Chapter Eight addresses the concept of *Spiritual Reflection* and encourages looking inside oneself to find peace, hope, and direction during difficult times, thereby exploring humanness as a whole: body, mind, and spirit.

Chapter Nine focuses on the *Days After Pregnancy Bedrest* and getting back on one's feet, as well as facing issues surrounding *Postpartum Depression*. This chapter provides education related to the different types of postpartum issues experienced by a woman after childbirth, along with recognizing symptoms of postpartum depression and developing coping strategies. Support contacts are provided for those seeking help.

Resources are a woman's best friend when trying to fill the many days that come with pregnancy bedrest. Appendix A provides a list of books, movie rental websites, newspaper websites, product sites for baby and mother, as well as much more.

In Appendix B, Kick count charts are provided for gestational weeks 28-40 to help the expectant mother monitor her unborn child's movements on a daily basis. Most OB/GYN's encourage monitoring the baby's movements during the last few months of pregnancy to ensure the baby is developing well. Not only does a kick count chart help to keep the doctor informed, it provides peace of mind for the expectant parents.

Chapter One

Author's Pregnancy Bedrest Memoir

൶൶൶൶൶൶൶൶൶൶

It's been seven and a half years since I was prescribed my first stint of pregnancy bedrest, and when I reflect back on the news, "You are going to spend the rest of your pregnancy in bed" I still feel nausea. What a journey! When deciding to share my personal stories about bedrest, I struggled with how detailed I should be about my experiences. Initially, I left out parts I thought might be frightening to women facing a lengthy bedrest experience. However, my husband, who is also my confidant, informed me I was not giving a realistic view of pregnancy bedrest. His comment, "By attempting to protect women from the difficult truths of bedrest, you are only perpetuating the attitude of bedrest not being a difficult experience, and it is for a lot of women and their families, as you know." I love him for his honesty. So, I will attempt to give all the facts as I remember them – the positive, the negative, and the in-between stage.

My goal is to encourage women to view bedrest as a journey of love while attempting to give their unborn baby every opportunity at life and health. While no woman would choose to go on bedrest, it's a sacrifice many of us have made - know you are not alone in this journey. Many women have come before you, others will come after you, and many are sharing the experience with you at this moment in time. This is your journey so embark on it the best you can, and the rest will come. A woman's attitude about her life situation plays a big role in the strength she has to draw from when faced with a crisis. Therefore, my challenge to you is to allow yourself to be who you are and to use this journey to grow – not just survive. The following stories are my personal experiences with bedrest. I hope they bring encouragement to your life.

1st Pregnancy Experience

After being married for nine years, my husband, Jon, and I began trying to conceive a pregnancy – fertility was not my friend. We struggled with fertility issues for about two years before I finally became pregnant. The words, "Wanda you're going to have a baby" were the sweetest words my doctor could have spoken.   I recall getting the news while Jon was at work, so my dog and I did a little victory dance for defeating the infertility monster. I chose to wait until Jon came home from work before telling him because I wanted to see the excitement on his face. That evening we shared tears as we had done so many evenings before; however, this time they were tears of joy. We were on our way to becoming parents!

The first trimester brought with it excitement and challenge.   I had morning sickness, what felt like twenty four hours per day, seven days per week, for approximately eight weeks. Working full time as a marriage and family therapist, I found it a struggle just to get to my office each day.   In addition to the morning sickness, I battled issues with low progesterone levels.   In an attempt to avoid a miscarriage, my doctor prescribed progesterone suppositories for daily use during the first trimester. Around sixteen weeks gestation things started looking up. The morning sickness subsided and my progesterone levels became normal.   Finally, I was feeling great and enjoying being pregnant.

Then, on February 12, 1998 (twenty-two weeks and two days gestation), I went to work just like all the other mornings. Several people at work commented, "Wanda you are glowing; you look so cute pregnant." I was glowing - inside and out! The most precious gift in the world was going to be mine very soon. I went into session with a client that morning feeling fine and being aware of my baby being active. Upon completing the session, I felt a strong urge to urinate. When I went to the restroom, I discovered I was bleeding and had lost my mucous plug. The fear that gripped my heart during that moment will be with me forever – I felt that I couldn't breath. Composing myself the best I could, I returned to my office to telephone my doctor. I was so shaken that it took four attempts at dialing the number before I got it correct. My doctor told me to go straight to the hospital and she would meet me in the labor and delivery hall.

Because I felt too distressed to drive, a colleague drove me to Jon's office and he, in turn, drove me to the hospital. When I looked into my husband's eyes, I could see the fear. He tried to comfort me on the way to the hospital, but we both knew my situation was not good. Upon arriving at the hospital, I was taken to labor and delivery and was assessed for blood loss and was monitored for contractions and the baby's heartbeat. My doctor arrived and performed an ultrasound and a manual exam, from which she discovered the placenta was lying close to the cervix. I had expelled my mucous plug, dilated 1 cm, and was contracting every two minutes. The diagnosis was preterm labor caused by placenta previa. To

12

say I was scared out of my mind was an understatement. My doctor reassured me the baby was doing fine, but my uterus was being defiant.

With my being only twenty-two weeks pregnant, my doctor was concerned about early deliver. Her calm presence was a blessing during those moments of crisis. She took my hand and placed it between both of hers and said, "Wanda, your situation is very serious, and I can't make you any promises except I will do everything I can to help you and your baby." The tears I cried at that moment were from the deepest part of my soul. My heart felt it was physically aching and the fear was overwhelming.

The questions began: Why is this happening to me? How will I go on if my baby dies? Did I do something to cause this to occur? The questions in my mind were endless, and the feelings in my heart immeasurable. Fear, sadness, guilt, anger, and grief, among other emotions, were all circulating through my heart and mind.

After blood test results and several hours of monitoring contractions and the baby's heartbeat, my doctor broke the pregnancy bedrest news. She said I would need to remain in the hospital until the bleeding subsided and the contractions slowed. Once things were under control I would be placed on strict bedrest with only bathroom privileges. If my baby were to have a strong chance of surviving, I would need to attain twenty-eight weeks gestation, with the ultimate goal being thirty-six weeks. She informed me I was to have intravenous medication: Magnesium Sulfate, which would help get the contractions and bleeding under control. I recall her saying, "Wanda, this medication is no fun but it is necessary – hang in there; you can do it."

Once my doctor left, a nurse came in and hooked me up to the Magnesium Sulfate, and within minutes, I felt horrible. Hot flashes, nausea, vomiting, inability to concentrate, and lack of movement were the symptoms I most recall - not to mention the agony of the Folley Catheter that comes with the medication. I remember lying in the hospital bed thinking, "How can this be happening to us?" Everything seemed to be happening so fast that I was unable to wrap my mind around the whole picture. It wasn't long before I started the bargaining process in my mind and heart with God. I really struggled with self blame. Intellectually, I knew my pregnancy condition was the result of an unpreventable medical complication. However, emotionally and spiritually I needed to blame someone, so I blamed myself.

Later that night, my doctor visited and let me know things were looking better. The bleeding was decreasing and the Magnesium Sulfate seemed to be helping with the contractions. After forty-eight hours on Magnesium Sulfate, I was transitioned to oral Terbutaline. Finally, the bleeding stopped and the contractions greatly decreased. On day five, I was considered stable enough to return home. Strict pregnancy bedrest with bathroom privileges was my prescription, along with 2.5 mg of Terbutaline to be taken every four hours.

Over the next three weeks, I visited the hospital for scheduled intravenous medications. The visits were scheduled for a 24 hour stay; however, they usually lasted from 48 to 72 hours. For some unknown reason, the medications slightly stimulated my contractions, raising medical concerns. To be safe rather than sorry, I would stay in the hospital until my contractions stabilized. As for the oral Terbutaline, it worked for several weeks in keeping the contractions at bay.

In addition to oral Terbutaline, I performed home uterine monitoring twice daily. After monitoring for an hour, a home health care nurse would call and report how I was doing. These reports provided a sense of relief. In the back of my mind was the constant thought of the contractions increasing and of my baby being born too early. Having a uterine monitoring device available to me around the clock brought a sense of peace and control to my life.

While my bedrest situation was not welcomed with open arms, I was more fortunate than many women in the same situation. My in-laws, Shirley and Earl, were kind enough to put their lives on hold for fourteen weeks and take care of us. I felt blessed to have family that could and would make such a sacrifice for our unborn baby. Shirley did all the cooking and cleaning. Earl cared for the lawn and other things around the house, as well as being my daily "Price is Right" viewing partner. We had great fun – he's much better at estimating prices than I.

During the first few weeks of bedrest, I was able to keep myself busy by learning about my medical condition and keeping weekly hospital visits. Around week five, however, I started feeling the physical and emotional effects of bedrest. As a result of lying on my sides constantly, the joints in my legs and arms became sore and painful. In addition to joint pain, my head hurt from the medication and constant heartburn was terrible. Boredom was also beginning to set in. Not having experienced bedrest before, I was ill equipped with what to do to entertain myself for lengthy periods of time. And, honestly, there were days when all I wanted to do was lie in bed and feel sorry for myself – entertainment wasn't even a thought. However, on my good days, I read, watched television, called friends, wrote letters, and did anything I could do to keep my mind off my pregnancy complications.

Things seemed to be going well up until week twenty-nine. During my 29th week of pregnancy, contractions increased, bringing about another trip to the hospital. Upon arriving at the hospital, the nurse began monitoring my contractions and the baby's heartbeat. The contractions were two minutes apart and strong. The dreaded news came that I had to be put on Magnesium Sulfate again. Apparently, I had habituated to the oral Terbutaline and the only course of action was Magnesium Sulfate. This time, it was for four days at relatively high doses.

Once the contractions seemed to be under control again, I was transitioned off the Magnesium Sulfate onto a Terbutaline subcutaneous pump, a small machine that looked like a beeper. It hooked onto the waistband of my pants, and I wore it around the clock for continuous delivery of medication. This was the same kind of pump used with diabetic patients who need continuous insulin delivery; however, the medication was Terbutaline.

After two days of working with the Terbutaline pump and getting the dosage correct, I was released to go home. Home health nurses came to visit the day I returned home to educate me about the pump, including how to clean the site, change the medication syringe, change the needle, and how to insert the needle into my thigh – myself! I was not too cool with my new nursing duties because needles frighten me. Fortunately, Jon was not squeamish around needles, so he cleaned the site and changed the needle every third day. However, there was one occasion I had to change the needle myself. I had taken a shower, and while drying off, I accidentally pulled the needle out of my thigh. "Panicked" is the word that comes to mind to describe my feelings. I knew I could not go without the medication and Jon was at work. I called him on the telephone and said, "You have to come home right away; the needle came out of my thigh!" He was in a meeting and could not leave, so I had to play nurse to myself. After about four attempts, I actually broke the skin and inserted the needle. While to most, this would seem nothing to get upset about, for me it seemed an overwhelming task. This was just one more undesired thing I endured to make it through the pregnancy. That same night, I remember telling Jon, "I don't think I can do this anymore." By this time, I had been in bed for two months and struggling with what felt was every aspect of my being.

Maintaining my sanity at times felt almost impossible. My feelings were mixed - I loved that I was wonderfully created to bring forth life - a beautiful baby my heart so desired. However, the flip side was that I felt angry at my wonderfully created body because it seemed to be failing me when I needed it most. I felt as though everything in my life had changed in a moment. In essence it did. I struggled with feeling isolated, anxious, worried, angry, and at times, somewhat depressed. The journey seemed endless and I was miserable.

Fortunately, I had a moment of clarity in my thinking and realized I had to change my attitude about being in bed if I were to be sane when all was said and done. I knew I had, somehow, to take back some control and not continue to be a victim of pregnancy bedrest. I needed to start living instead of just surviving. How to begin was the million dollar question. It didn't take long to figure out I needed openly to grieve and to find acceptance in my current life situation. I had suffered a great loss, and I was not addressing it. My attitude was terrible, and I did nothing but complain. Not being able to control what was happing with my pregnancy, left me feeling completely out of control in life. My goal changed from trying to survive bedrest from day to day, to turning my obstacles into opportunities. Lying in bed, paralyzed with fear about what could happen, was stealing the joy I had once felt about becoming a mother. While I could not control the physical aspects of pregnancy, I could control how I was responding to my pregnancy and work on restoring my joy and lessen my mental anguish.

Focusing on the positive aspects of my journey and positive self talk was how I planned to turn things around. I began by journaling my feelings on a daily basis. Journaling was a great outlet for anger, grief, fear, anxiety, depression, and other emotions. Writing my thoughts and feelings on paper provided a sense of relief. As far as my daily activities, I began to read more, do more puzzles, write more letters, telephone friends more frequently, and watch more movies – anything to keep my mind off being in bed and worrying about the baby. Being able to speak with friends and discuss issues outside of my situation was great! Often times, our conversations would bring laughter along with a little gossip. These conversations were beneficial in helping me to feel a sense of connection to the world outside of the bedroom and bathroom. When the negative thoughts crept into my mind, I acknowledged they were there and made a conscious choice to think of what was going right in my life. Positive thinking made a big difference in my outlook on the rest of my pregnancy and brought with it hope and peace.

Another dimension of my new attitude was spending more quality time with Jon in the evenings. We had spent a great deal of time together every evening; however, most of it was listening to me complain about being on bedrest, worrying about the baby, and enduring physical pain. Don't tell him, but I think I was a LITTLE jealous of his freedom. We began to express our fears, desires, plans, and hopes as a couple who were experiencing bedrest, instead of just focusing on my misery. When I reflect on my self-indulgence of distress, I feel somewhat negligent in being supportive of Jon's feelings. However, he was a champ in giving me what I needed – time! The time did come when I was able to be there for him and to understand how our situation was affecting both of us. Having a more positive focus in the midst of our crisis was the fuel we needed for our journey. I consciously reminded myself that "this is his baby also, and he is afraid." Reminding myself, "I'm not alone" helped to make the days, hours, and at times, minutes more manageable. Some of my fondest memories were of when we snuggled up in bed to watch movies, play games, share our thoughts, and enjoy my favorite activity - playing poker for M&M's. While I did not have gestational diabetes, my diet was restricted because of the medications. By the time I had completed bedrest, I was ready for a trip to Las Vegas – my poker skills had increased immensely. Jon should have known never to stand between a pregnant woman and her chocolate!

The change in attitude was exactly what I needed to restore the joy I had once felt about becoming a mother. I still had bad days, but I chose not to stay stuck in them. Eventually, the good outweighed the bad and I was finally living and not just surviving. At thirty-six weeks gestation, I went in to see the doctor for my weekly visit, and she released me from bedrest. I felt as a person probably feels after being released from incarceration for a lengthy time. I felt free once again. All medication was discontinued, no more uterine monitoring necessary, and I was encouraged to "resume normal activities." I was so excited! I couldn't wait to dine in my favorite Chinese restaurant and go shopping for baby things. What I failed to realize was that after lying in bed for fourteen weeks the spirit may want to go but the body says, "slow down." By the time I showered, dressed, styled my hair and applied make-up, I had to lie down and rest before going out. After walking from the car into the restaurant, consuming food vertically as opposed to horizontally, and walking back to the car, my only desire was to get home and rest. I didn't realize how much my muscle strength and physical endurance level had been depleted during this fourteen week time frame - I was exhausted!

Later, after my first outing, contractions picked up and I, again, went to the hospital. Upon arriving at the hospital, I was admitted to deliver our baby. My contractions were five minutes apart and my cervix had dilated to 2cm. The long awaited day had arrived. I was both scared and excited. I was physically wiped out; however, my heart and soul were full of excitement and anticipation about the gift I would be holding in just a few hours. After blood work was completed, I received an epidural and the waiting began. Because my labor was not progressing, my bag of water was broken and Pitocin started. After about thirteen hours of labor, I was rushed in for an emergency c-section. The baby's heartbeat started dipping lower with each contraction. All went well with the c-section and Lydia was born. She weighed 5 pounds and 5 ounces. I got to see her long enough to kiss her on the head before she was whisked off to the nursery to be evaluated.

Upon awaking in recovery, I was panicked. For some reason, I thought Lydia had died. The nurse finally convinced me to calm down and wheeled my bed by the nursery so I could see my beautiful daughter. I cried once again; however, this time the tears were of joy and peace. We had made it! My little girl was healthy and breathing on her own. A miracle took place in my life that night.

While bedrest was no walk in the park and the days after Lydia's birth were somewhat challenging physically, I grew in ways I never dreamed possible. The pregnancy bedrest experience left me with the feeling that there is nothing I couldn't accomplish if I really put my mind to it. One of the many things I learned about myself is I am truly a blessed woman with strengths previously unbeknown to me. My outcome was perfect, and I am grateful for that everyday of my life. My daughter Lydia is now seven years old and is healthy in all aspects - she is beautiful, smart, sweet, and will someday be a strong woman.

2nd Pregnancy Experience

After having a difficult time conceiving Lydia, Jon and I were unsure if we would ever experience the miracle of life again. To our surprise, we were able to conceive a second pregnancy without fertility issues. Upon finding out I was pregnant for a second time, my feelings were somewhat mixed - excited about the possibility of another child, and frightened about the possibility of another stint of pregnancy bedrest and this time with a toddler.

Prior to my second pregnancy, we relocated to another city, which mandated I had to find a new OB/GYN. Commuting to my previous doctor's office was not recommended for someone with my pregnancy history. At first, I felt somewhat uncomfortable with this change; however, my new doctor was wonderful and he specialized in high risk obstetrics. During my first appointment, I explained how things went during my first pregnancy, and he was very clear in stating that I would likely end up in bed with my second pregnancy as well. I knew this in the back of my mind; however, hearing him say it made the inevitable more real. He encouraged me to limit my lifting, to rest as much as possible, and try not to worry. When Jon and I left his office that afternoon, I remember asking, "How will I do bedrest and care for Lydia?"

Upon arriving home from the doctor's office, Jon called his parents and let them know we would possibly need their help again. Fortunately, they were able and willing to commit to helping us if need be; they are amazing people!

During the first trimester, the pregnancy unfolded similar to my pregnancy with Lydia, except for the low progesterone level, which was normal this time around. I was no longer working outside of the home, so, fortunately, I was able to rest and relax. Knowing bedrest could be just around the corner, I began taking the necessary precautions. When Lydia napped, I napped with her, and I was able to limit my lifting by moving her to a toddler bed, as well as taking care of things I knew would be coming up in the next few months. I could do nothing more than just wait and hope things would be different this time. Although I tried not to worry, worry was impossible. In my heart, I knew I would be on bedrest again.

As I began approaching the twenty week time frame, I couldn't help wondering how things would go this time. If I went on bedrest, would I be as fortunate this time as I was the last time with having a health baby? I knew I could do it again; it was not knowing the outcome that created stress for me. Then, on August 25, 2000 (twenty-two weeks and five days gestation) I felt the contractions begin. I called my doctor's office and he requested I come in for contraction and baby heartbeat monitoring. Before leaving the house, I sat with Lydia on my lap for a few minutes and held her close. "How will she feel if I have to stay in bed and will she feel less loved?" were the questions running through my mind. We sat for a few minutes, and then off we went to the doctor's office. Jon met up with me so he could take care of Lydia while I was being monitored. He took my hand and said, "Wanda, we can do this if we have to; remember it's worth it – here's our proof, and he held up Lydia." When he spoke those words, I knew we would be okay – I wasn't alone.

Sure enough, I was having contractions from placenta previa once again, but minimal dilation, and no bleeding this time. The diagnosis was preterm labor with low lying placenta. I was permitted to return home that same day with my course of treatment being strict bedrest with bathroom privileges and Procardia to prevent contractions.

Upon arriving home, Jon called his parents to let them know I was on pregnancy bedrest again. They were wonderful! They jumped in their car the next morning and were at our house before we knew it. I don't know what we would have done without them.

19

While the first twenty two weeks of my second pregnancy were very similar to the first pregnancy, the bedrest experience was quite a bit different. I did frequent the hospital on several occasions for increasing contractions; however, I did not have to endure the Magnesium Sulfate nor any overnight stays. When my contractions increased, I went to the hospital for monitoring and receiving a Terbutaline shot before returning home. Avoiding lengthy hospital stays was a nice change from the previous experience.

Another significant difference from the first experience was that I had a two year old to care for during this stint of bedrest. It wasn't just about Jon and me this time around, but also about Lydia. My goal was to get all of us, my unborn baby, Lydia, and me through this bedrest journey as unscathed as possible.

Mindful of my past pregnancy bedrest experience, I worked hard at not allowing negative thinking to creep into my mind. When I got into a self-defeating mode of thinking, I turned my focus to Lydia and remembered she was my proof that the difficult journey of pregnancy bedrest is nothing compared to the prize – my daughter. Many times I felt I was running on empty – caring for Lydia from bed (as much as was permitted), abiding by doctor's orders, dealing with gestational diabetes, battling physical pain and emotional distress, as well as suffering the side effects from medication. I certainly had my moments of thinking, "Will this journey every end?"

As the thirty-six week gestation time approached, I could hardly contain my excitement. I wanted nothing more than to get out of bed and walk around. At thirty-six weeks, once again, I was released into the free world. All medication was discontinued, and I was encouraged to return to my normal activities. This time I was much smarter about "returning to my normal activities." I took life very slowly. On the fifth day, after coming off bedrest, my water broke and off to the hospital we went. I was very excited. Finally, my day had arrived. After eight hours of labor, I was holding my precious, healthy little boy. Caleb weighed 7 pounds and 3 ounces. Once again, I felt like the most blessed woman in the world. I now had both a beautiful girl and a handsome boy.

As with the first bedrest experience, physical recovery took awhile, but I am pleased to report we are all healthy and doing great. Caleb is a sweet, smart, energetic four year old little boy who has become a huge part of our hearts. When I look at my children, my heart is full of love, and when I think about my gestational journeys with them, I am proud of the woman and mother I have become. I now know life is a journey, and our experiences make us who we are and influence who we will become.

Chapter Two

Medical Reasons for Pregnancy Bedrest
Different Types of Pregnancy Bedrest
Questions for Your Doctor

ঔ৶ ঔ৶ ঔ৶ ঔ৶ ঔ৶ ঔ৶ ঔ৶ ঔ৶ ঔ৶ ঔ৶

From the time we, as women, begin thinking about having a child, we tend to paint a portrait in our minds about how our pregnancy journey will unfold. We focus on how to decorate the nursery, we anticipate shopping for baby clothes, having baby shower fun, being adored by others as our girth expands, and many other joys associated with pregnancy. Unfortunately, for some women, the portrait does not depict how the journey actually takes place: lying in bed for weeks, if not months, on end.

When complications arise during pregnancy, an OB/GYN often times prescribes pregnancy bedrest with the goal of helping both mother and baby having every opportunity for life and health. While no woman wants to hear the dreaded words, "You have to go on bedrest" most women understand bedrest can be an opportunity for their unborn child.

It's important to note that pregnancy bedrest does not guarantee a perfect outcome and is considered by some in the medical community a controversial form of treatment because of health issues that can result from lying in bed for extended periods of time and questions as to the effectiveness of bedrest in preventing premature births. While there is controversy surrounding the prescription of bedrest, many physicians still prescribe bedrest because they believe it can possibly help a threatened pregnancy and hopefully delay delivery. The belief is that when lying in a reclined position, pressure from the baby is taken off the cervix and this reduction in pressure may possibly reduce the stretching of the cervix, which, in turn, may decrease the chances of contractions, miscarriage, preterm labor, rupture of membranes, and/or vaginal bleeding. Bedrest may also increase oxygen and nutrients delivery to the baby when it is growing poorly due to problems with the placenta. Bedrest may also help the mother's organs function more efficiently by improving heart and kidney function, as well as helping with the management of high blood pressure and swelling. Additionally, a decrease in activity and an increase in rest may help in reducing uterine irritability, contractions, and possibly bleeding for some women.

In this chapter, I will take the opportunity, briefly, to mention and describe some of the medical conditions under which pregnancy bedrest might be prescribed, discuss various types of pregnancy bedrest, and to pose questions for your doctor. Please keep in mind, I am not a physician, and am in no way attempting to diagnose or treat pregnancy conditions. Should you have "any" questions or concerns pertaining to your pregnancy condition, or your personal health, contact your doctor for support.

Medical reasons for pregnancy bedrest

The following medical conditions can possibly lead the expectant mother to pregnancy bedrest. Please note preterm labor as listed first with possible causes; however, not every woman experiencing these preterm labor "precursors" will actually experience preterm labor, but these conditions can bring on preterm labor.

- *Preterm Labor*: A woman is believed to be in preterm labor if she begins having regular contractions that cause changes to the cervix (opening, thinning, or shortening) prior to 37 weeks gestation. Preterm labor often presents with one or more of the following symptoms: lower back pain, diarrhea, tightening sensation in the abdomen (may feel like the baby is balling up), stomach cramps, pelvic pressure, and vaginal discharge. Some preterm labor is unexplained and no particular medical cause can be determined. However, most preterm labor is brought about by some type(s) of medical condition(s), such as bacterial vaginosis, incompetent cervix, premature rupture of membranes, placenta previa, preeclampsia, intrauterine growth retardation, and multiple gestation.

  Bedrest may be beneficial for the woman experiencing preterm labor by reducing activity, which hopefully will help with the reduction in contractions, bleeding, and cervical dilation.

- *Bacterial Vaginosis*: Bacterial vaginosis results from an overgrowth of normal bacteria found in the vagina, a condition known as a genital tract infection. This condition is characterized by an abnormal vaginal discharge and/or foul odor. Because some women never experience these symptoms, they do not realize they have bacterial vaginosis until it shows up in pregnancy. It is believed that bacterial vaginosis in pregnancy can bring on preterm labor and possibly infection of the amniotic fluid. Reducing physical activities may help prevent and/or reduce contractions and, perhaps, delay labor until this condition can be treated with medications.

- *Incompetent Cervix*: Incompetent cervix is diagnosed when the cervix begins to open too early in pregnancy. The cervix should stay tightly closed until the right time for the baby to be born. This condition is often treated with a cerclage, which is a small stitch placed in the cervix to prevent further opening. Most women with a diagnosis of an incompetent cervix will spend time in bed since lying down may reduce pressure placed on the cervix, hopefully, helping to keep the cervix closed until the appropriate time for delivery.

- *Premature Rupture of Membranes (PROM)*: Premature rupture of membranes (PROM) is characterized by a gush and/or a constant dribble of fluid from the vagina as a result of the membranes surrounding the baby rupturing too early in the pregnancy.

PROM is a serious pregnancy medical condition that must be assessed immediately by an OB/GYN or health care provider. Contractions usually accompany PROM which puts the baby at great risk for early delivery. In some cases, the doctor can hold off delivery with medications; however, if the medications do not work, the baby is usually born within twenty-four to seventy-two hours. Some cases of PROM are unexplained, however, some occur because of the following conditions: more than one baby is developing in the uterus; excessive amount of amniotic fluid known as hydramnios; incompetent cervix; bacterial infection of one or more reproductive organs; preterm labor with contractions and/or cervical dilation; and physical injury – accidental or domestic violence.

The goal of pregnancy bedrest with PROM patients is to decrease contractions as much as possible, as well as to prevent cervical dilation. Every day is important when faced with delivering a preterm baby. If the baby is responding in a healthy manner, even though the membranes have ruptured, a doctor may put a woman on bedrest hoping to get as much growth time as possible for the baby.

- *Placenta Previa*: Placenta previa usually becomes apparent with painless, bright red bleeding from the vagina. This condition occurs when the placenta is not implanted high in the uterus but is located very close to the cervix (within centimeters), partially on the cervix, or completely covering the cervix. No episodes of bleeding, one episode, or numerous episodes of bleeding, depending on the severity of the previa, may be present.

  Placenta previa is a serious complication and is almost always treated with strict bedrest. The good news is that placenta previa often corrects itself as the uterus grows. Uterine growth can allow the placenta to move away from the cervix. When the placenta previa does not correct itself, a c-section may be necessary to keep the mother and the baby out of harm's way. However, a normal vaginal delivery is certainly possible if the previa corrects itself and if there are no other problems. The majority of babies born to mothers experiencing placenta previa have very good outcomes.

  Most doctors prescribe pregnancy bedrest for placenta previa in hopes of reducing and/or preventing vaginal bleeding, increase oxygen and nutrient delivery to the baby, stop or decrease contractions, and prevent premature birth.

- *Preeclampsia*: Preeclampsia, also known as toxemia, presents with high blood pressure, swelling of the legs, hands, face and/or of the entire body, plus protein in the urine. Eclampsia is a complication of preeclampsia marked by seizures or coma. Expectant mothers with a preeclampsia diagnosis are monitored closely in the hope of getting the condition under control. Preeclampsia can prevent the placenta from getting enough blood, thereby, decreasing oxygen and nutrient delivery to the baby. As a result of the reduction in oxygen and nutrients to the uterus, the baby may experience low birth weight and other problems.

With a diagnosis of preeclampsia, the OB/GYN may prescribe bedrest in an attempt to decrease blood pressure, swelling, and protein in the urine, as well as increasing oxygen and nutrient delivery to the baby. Taking weight off the woman's large blood vessels, bodily function increases for both baby and mother.

- *Intrauterine Growth Retardation (IUGR)*: Intrauterine Growth Retardation (IUGR) is diagnosed when the baby is growing more slowly than is normal and is smaller than it should be for its gestational age. IUGR can be brought about by numerous factors such as hazardous chemical exposure, alcohol, drug and/or tobacco use by the mother, maternal health problems such as diabetes, heart disease, hypertension, sexually transmitted diseases, and autoimmune deficiency diseases, pregnancy conditions such as placenta previa, gestational diabetes, multiple gestation, and preeclampsia, maternal mental health issues such as anorexia and bulimia, and from genetic and chromosomal disorders suffered by the baby.

The goal of pregnancy bedrest for IUGR is to try and prevent premature delivery and increase oxygen and nutrient delivery to the baby while allowing every opportunity for growth. Many cases exist in which there is no explanation for the IUGR pregnancy. In cases where there are explanations such as anorexia, bulimia, drug abuse, alcoholism, and tobacco use, it's important to stop these behaviors immediately and to follow your doctor's orders. If help is needed in abstaining from these harmful behaviors, please ask your doctor to point out a professional who can help!

While it would be normal to worry about a baby's lack of growth, remember that doesn't necessarily mean he/she will suffer from disabilities. Talk with your doctor about any concerns and follow his or her advice.

- *Multiple Gestation*: Multiple gestation is a pregnancy consisting of two or more babies. Multiple gestation pregnancies tend to have a higher risk of complications related to pre-term labor, incompetent cervix, premature rupture of membranes (PROM), preeclampsia, and intrauterine growth retardation (IUGR).

When prescribing bedrest for multiple gestation, the goal is to help prevent preterm delivery as long as possible to allow each baby to get to a safe weight and healthy stage of development before birth. A decrease in activity may aid in lowering blood pressure and swelling, allowing the body to deliver oxygen and nutrients more efficiently to the baby. Also, bedrest may help the mother's organs to function more efficiently.

If diagnosed with one or more of the above conditions, be sure to get all the information needed from your doctor. Education can bring with it a sense of control in a situation that can seem out of control. Unanswered questions can lead to misunderstanding a diagnosis, as well as to an increase in stress and anxiety. Each woman owes herself, her partner, her family, and her unborn baby to have questions answered.

The next point of focus in this writing is the various types of pregnancy bedrest. The most common pregnancy bedrest prescriptions are partial (modified), strict, and complete (hospital). The information presented here is to provide an idea of what each type of bedrest entails. Doctors will have a specific plan for each type of pregnancy bedrest, so follow your doctor's orders. Do not alter bedrest orders based on information presented here or elsewhere.

Different types of pregnancy bedrest

- *Partial or Modified Bedrest*: Being prescribed partial or modified bedrest may mean spending at least part of the day lying down and resting on the sofa or bed. Depending on the seriousness of a pregnancy's complications, a doctor may allow the woman to be up several hours and possibly work from home or perform other activities at home not considered a threat to the pregnancy condition. Modified bedrest could range from a few hours in bed per day to a stricter bedrest routine allowing only a few hours out of bed per day. Restrictions from sexual intercourse, exercise, and lifting may be a part of the modified bedrest routine. Nail down the specifics with your doctor, so that there is no confusion pertaining to limitations.

- *Strict Bedrest*: When prescribed, strict bedrest means exactly as it sounds. Time out of bed will certainly be limited. Most strict bedrest patients are allowed only shower and bathroom privileges. Some will have the privilege of sitting while eating, while others will be required to remain in a reclined position even during meals. Depending on the seriousness of the pregnancy condition, the woman may be able to shower daily and to make as many trips to the bathroom as necessary. However, some strict bedrest patients will only be permitted to shower every other day and be given a limited number of trips to the bathroom. If bathroom privileges are restricted, the patient will be required to use a bedpan. As with modified bedrest, strict bedrest patients are encouraged to abstain from sexual intercourse, exercise, lifting, and activities that could worsen the pregnancy condition. Again, it is very important to know the exact limitations of your pregnancy bedrest prescription.

- *Complete or Hospital Bedrest*: Obviously, complete or hospital bedrest is the most severe type of bedrest. When a woman is prescribed complete bedrest, she will likely have to spend time in a hospital. She may be prescribed complete bedrest because her pregnancy condition is serious enough that continual monitoring by a health care specialist is required. These women will use a bedpan for bathroom privileges and provided hygiene services by hospital staff, unless a family member is able and willing to perform those services. Some woman will even have a catheter in place. Trendelenburg positioning may also be required for some patients experiencing complete bedrest. Trendelenburg positioning is placing the patient's head lower than the rest of the body to alleviate pressure on the cervix. Again, complete bedrest patients are encouraged to abstain from sexual intercourse, exercise, and activities that could worsen the pregnancy condition.

The three types of bedrest listed above are the most common; however, a doctor may modify each one based on the woman's particular needs. It's important that all pregnant woman on bedrest understand what medicines have been prescribed and what activities are allowed. I cannot stress enough the importance of this knowledge.

Another important factor to consider when placed on bedrest, especially one that is strict or complete, is circulation issues. Speak with your doctor about possible exercises to prevent blood clots and lessen muscle pain and strain. Inactivity may certainly be advantageous to a complicated pregnancy situation; however, it brings with it some disadvantages. These disadvantages can include muscle and joint pain, muscle weakness, blood clots, headaches as a result of poor circulation, and dizziness. Discuss the possibility of a physical therapy plan with your OB/GYN for your pregnancy condition. <u>I do not encourage any exercises prior to speaking with a doctor, even the ones presented in this book.</u>

While bedrest may seem like a mountain that is insurmountable, trust me – the challenge is achievable. The inner strength of a woman, you, in particular, is awesome. Being a mother might mean you have to make concessions from time to time; however, these concessions may be necessary in helping your baby to have every opportunity at life. There will be days when you think "I cannot stay in this bed for one more minute." However, allow yourself some bad days and just try not to get stuck in those moments of distress; better days are ahead.

Also, keep in mind that when diagnosed with a high risk pregnancy it is crucial to know exactly what activities are permitted and what activities are not permitted. This will help with planning your bedrest days. I have compiled a list of questions to pose to your OB/GYN. The questions listed here are ones I had personally, as well as questions other women have had when faced with pregnancy bedrest. Remember, ask your doctor any question for which an answer is needed. Knowing exactly what can and cannot be done while on bedrest will bring feelings of relaxation and a sense of control. Also, remember there are no stupid questions. You, your baby, and family are the most important factors to focus on during this time, so any question deserves an answer.

Questions for your doctor

Q: How much time will I have to stay in bed per day?
A: _____

Q: How much time will I be allowed out of bed per day?
A: _____

Q: When in bed, what position is best: sitting-up, reclined, or left side?
A: _____

Q: Does my time out of bed mean I can walk around, or is this time allowed only to eat, shower, change clothes, etc.?
A: _____

Q: Will I be allowed to shower daily?
A: _____

Q: Is there a time limit on how long I can be in the shower?
A: _____

Q: Will I need to sit on a shower chair while showering, or can I stand?
A: _____

Q: Will I be allowed to take a tub bath?
A: _____

Q: If I cannot shower daily, will I be allowed time to wash up quickly on non-shower days? How much time can I dedicate to washing up on non-shower days?
A: _____

Q: Can I get up to use the bathroom when I feel it is necessary, or will my trips to the bathroom be limited, thus requiring use of a bedpan?
A: _____

Q: Will I be allowed to continue to work?
A: _____

Q: If allowed to work, will the time be the same as my regular office or home work hours?
A: _____

Q: How much time can I daily sit in an upright position?
A: _____

Q: Will I be permitted to drive my car? If not, why not?
A: _____

Q: What possible medications will be prescribed for my pregnancy condition, and what reactions to those medications can I expect?
A: _____
_____
_____

Q: Will the pregnancy medications interact with other medications I have to take for other health conditions? If so, how?
A: _____
_____

Q: How much and how often will I need to take the prescribed medications?

A: _____

Q: If taking medication that causes a drop in blood pressure, what should I do if I feel faint or dizzy?

A: _____

Q: What over the counter medications are safe for me to take should I experience a headache, indigestion, constipation, cold, etc?

A: _____
_____
_____
_____

Q: How much water should I consume on a daily basis?

A: _____

Q: Will I have diet restrictions? If yes, which foods should I avoid?

A: _____
_____
_____
_____

Q: Will I be allowed to exercise? If so, exactly what exercises will be safe for me to perform while on bedrest?

A: _____
_____
_____

Q: Will I be allowed to climb stairs while on bedrest?

A: _____

Q: Will I be allowed to perform any lifting activities? If yes, what types of lifting?

A: _____

Q: Will I be permitted to perform housework such as washing dishes, sweeping, etc.?

A: _____

Q: Can I prepare meals for my family?
A: _____

Q: Will I be permitted to attend school activities for my other children?
A: _____

Q: Will I be able to provide care for my other children, such as bathing and grooming them?
A: _____

Q: Will I be able to care for my pet?
A: _____

Q: Is sexual activity permitted?
A: _____

Q: Is stimulation of breasts in preparation for breastfeeding permitted?
A: _____

Q: Will I be allowed to attend child birthing classes? If not, are videos and/or written materials to use for educational purposes available?
A: _____

Q: If the doctor is running behind schedule, should I find somewhere to lie down, or is it okay for me to sit?
A: _____

Q: What is the acceptable threshold for contractions? How many per hour, as well as the length of time the contractions can be expected?
A: _____
_____

Q: If on medications that affect heart rate and blood pressure, what is the acceptable threshold for both heart rate and blood pressure?
A: _____
_____

Q: What specific physical symptoms should lead me to call the doctor?
A: _____
_____
_____

Q: If I have complications, and the doctor is unavailable, who will fill in for him or her?

A: _____

Q: If my water breaks, should I go straight to the hospital?

A: _____

Q: Where should I go first when going to the hospital – emergency room or labor and delivery?

A: _____

While this is not a comprehensive list of questions, it's a good starting point. Different questions will come up throughout the bedrest journey. Use the "Questions for Doctor" pad provided with the Pregnancy Bedrest Essentials set, which can also be purchased separately from www.PregnancyBedrestEssentials.com to keep track of your questions and thoughts. Remember, ask any question for which an answer is needed; knowledge is power. Also, if certain requirements are impossible to follow, tell your doctor. Together, the two of you may be able to devise a plan that will better suit your particular needs.

Chapter Three

Tips for Managing and Coping with Pregnancy Bedrest

❧❧❧❧❧❧❧❧❧❧

After arriving home from my first hospital stay for pregnancy bedrest, I remember lying in bed and thinking "Okay, what now?" I was at a loss as to what I was supposed to do other than stay in bed. The thought of bedrest had never entered my thinking, so I was unprepared to deal with the change. For the first few weeks, I watched television, talked on the telephone, read books, and looked at the clock. It wasn't long before I started feeling bored. Learning to fill my days while on bedrest was a challenge.

The goal of this chapter is to offer tips for managing and coping with the pregnancy bedrest journey both at home or in the hospital. I hope the following list of items, activities, and suggestions will help to fill your days and make bedrest more tolerable.

- Place an egg-crate sponge on top of your mattress to make it softer and more formable to your body. If your pregnancy medical condition requires overnight hospital stays, don't forget to take the egg-crate sponge with you to the hospital. Hospital beds become very uncomfortable after a few days.
- If your doctor permits, lying on a sofa, futon, or recliner can be options to lying on the bed.
- Select bedding that is comfortable and aesthetically pleasant.
- Select a couple of pillows for your head and neck, for back support when lying on your side, and for leg and arm support. It's not uncommon for legs and arms to hurt while lying for extended periods of time. A body pillow is a smart investment for bedrest and don't forget to take it to the hospital with you.
- Place a table or night stand directly beside the bed or sofa. You will need a place to put a drink, medication, clock, lamp, home

uterine monitoring system, telephone, snacks, books, and remote controls. A three drawer plastic stand is also good for storage.

- Have a folding lap table available for use during bedrest. This will provide a place for eating, writing, polishing nails, reading, activities with children, etc.
- Make sure your room temperature is at a comfortable level.
- A small refrigerator or ice chest can be a valuable possession near your resting place. This will allow for storage of food and drinks, as well as for medications that need to be kept cold. Some hospitals will permit patients to have a small refrigerator in their room.
- Ensure a lamp or ability for turning lights on/off when desired is available. (One of the "clapper" devices works well for keeping activity low and for still being able to control the lights.)
- Place a step stool by the bed. A step stool is especially helpful if the bed is very high. As time goes by and more weight is gained and muscle strength is lost, getting in and out of bed can become a task.
- Use a television with remote control and keep new batteries on hand.
- Utilizing a walkman or CD player with headphones is a good idea to drown out other noises, especially while in the hospital.
- Set up a computer beside the bed – a laptop is ideal and will help the days pass much faster while at home and/or in the hospital. If you do not have a computer, try to borrow one from a friend or try to rent one from an electronics store.
- Rent or buy an adult commode chair if the closest bathroom is upstairs – if in the hospital, a bedpan will be provided if needed.
- A shower chair is a valuable item as time passes and the legs get weaker. This item can be rented from a pharmaceutical supply store, or it can be purchased from local stores such as Wal-Mart and Target (one lady said she was able to borrow one from a local nursing home in her area.) This necessity may also be covered by your insurance company if your doctor writes an order for it. If in the hospital, the nursing staff will provide one for you if needed. I used mine frequently – even after the baby was born. Remember, once again, that it takes a while to get your leg strength back.
- Keep a telephone near the bed so you do not have to get up each time it rings. Make sure your answering machine is working, just

in case you do not feel like talking, but would like to return the call later. Also, try to call at least one person per day so that you continue to feel connected to the outside world. When using a telephone for financial transactions, remember to use a land line as opposed to a cordless telephone for security purposes. A telephone with speaker phone capabilities is great for the mother away from her child because of a hospital stay. A speaker phone allows the expectant mother to talk or to read a bedtime story to the child at home. This activity is good for young children or for children who do not like talking on the telephone.

- Assure that a water bottle is within arms reach and consume at least 12 glasses per day. Water is important for keeping the uterus hydrated and for reducing contractions. Additionally, water helps with the management of constipation.

- Place a small microwave in your room. Having a small microwave in the bedrest area will ensure having the option of a hot meal. Keep frozen dinners in an ice chest (cooler), take one out and put it in the microwave on the way to the bathroom, and on the way back to your bed retrieve the meal from the microwave. You will accomplish two tasks with one trip. Make sure your doctor is comfortable with your having microwave energy in your direct living space.

- Ensure that food, especially snacks, is close at hand. Nuts, peanut butter and crackers, cheese and crackers, boxed cereal, dried fruit, etc. are good snacks for bedrest patients.

- Keep medications in arms reach and since medication is within arms reach, remember to keep medications out of the reach of small children. If in the hospital, be sure you know exactly what medications your doctor has prescribed for you, the dosage of each medication, and how often you are to be administered each medication. Don't feel intimidated to ask questions pertaining to your care – you need to stay informed!

- Keep an alarm clock in arms reach since you may need to take medication during the night.

- Secure a lawn chair or camping cot for sunny, warm days when you may be permitted to lie on your deck, patio or lawn. Remember to check with your doctor first, making sure the extra activity is permitted for your pregnancy medical condition.

- Keep extra blankets and sheets on hand just in case you have a spill or need to change bedding.

- Keep extra clothes close by in case you have a spill or just want to change. Include pajamas, robe, slippers, under clothes, tops, pants, etc. Don't forget to wear a support bra during the day - your growing bust line needs the continual support.
- Keep the following close at hand: a box of tissues, lip balm, heartburn medication (only ones permitted by your doctor), ear plugs (it's difficult to sleep with nurses coming in and out of your room and other patient's doors slamming when in the hospital), and a sleep mask which will help with nap times if sensitive to light.
- Place a "knock before entering" sign on the hospital door handle to allow for some control over your privacy.
- Bring your own shampoo, conditioner, soap, toothpaste, and toilette paper to the hospital.
- Establish a daily routine. Having a daily routine will allow for a sense of normalcy to life.
  - Determine a morning wake up time and try to stick with it, but keep in mind there will be nights when rest doesn't come easy, and you may need to rest more the next day.
  - Try to eat all meals at the same time every day – of course there will be days when you get off schedule, but having a good routine in place for meal times will help with energy and rest.
  - If permitted to shower every day, then do so. If permitted to shower only every other day, splash cold water on your face during your trips to the bathroom and this will help with feeling refreshed.
  - Change out of pajamas every morning. Wearing regular clothes will make you feel less like a patient and more like your normal self. Do keep in mind comfortable clothing.
  - Continue to groom hair, nails, and skin as always.
  - If applying make-up is part of the daily routine, continue to do so. Remember to keep make-up remover cloths by the bed or on the back of the toilet to remove make-up each night.
  - Speak with your doctor about a daily exercise routine. The exercises provided in this book are specifically designed for bedrest patients; however, get your doctor's approval before starting any of these exercises.

- o Schedule two activities per day with the commitment of accomplishment in mind. At the end of the day, the woman who meets her activity goals will feel as if she did more than simply lie in bed all day – she will experience a sense of accomplishment.
- Identify activity limitations by talking with your doctor and write down these limitations. A good list of questions for your doctor is provided in Chapter Two.
- Use a baby monitor or bell to help get the attention of others without having to yell. If in the hospital, use the nurse call button, but keep in mind you are not the only patient and it may take a few minutes to get attention.
- Walkie-talkies were wonderful to have during my second bedrest stint. I was able to talk with my daughter each night while she was going to sleep. I was still a part of story time, prayer time, as well as singing her a lullaby while she was in her own bed.
- Have available baby books, magazines, catalogs, telephone book, address book, pregnancy books, crossword puzzles, or any type of materials that provide education, relaxation, and activity. These items can be stored in a backpack and placed by the bed for easy access.
- Keep wipes and cleansing cloths on hand. These are especially beneficial if spending time with a small child during the day.
- Keep toiletries close by including, a mirror, brush, comb, hair accessories, nail file, nail clippers, scissors, body lotion, make-up, tooth brush and tooth paste, mouthwash, deodorant, etc. These items can be placed in a plastic container so they are readily available when needed. Keeping all of these items in one container helps in keeping track of them both at home and in the hospital. Again, remember to keep small children safe from items that could cause harm.
- Keep paper, pencil, pen, stationery, and journal on hand. I found a backpack useful for storing these items as well as books and magazines. If small children are in the household, include markers, crayons, coloring books, story books, and other activities in the backpack as well.
- Place an ultrasound picture in a frame or tape it in an area where it is visible. Reminding yourself why you are undertaking the task of pregnancy bedrest will help keep you motivated.
- Notify neighbors of your situation just in case of an emergency. Also, you may want to ask a neighbor to sign for packages,

deliveries, and/or registered mail that might come while you are in bed.

- Collect menus from restaurants. Call local restaurants and request a mailed menu. Some restaurants deliver and, in cases where they don't, call ahead and have food waiting for someone to pick up and bring home. Also, local services may be available through Meals on Wheels for meals to be delivered to shut-ins. This is especially beneficial for bedrest patients who do not have someone cooking for them during the day. When in the hospital, let the nutritionist know what foods you like and dislike. Likely, the hospital will be willing to accommodate your wishes.

- Use your local library as a resource. Call your library and tell them you need books, tapes, etc. for the period while you are on bedrest. Most libraries will deliver to shut-ins and, if not, you can have someone bring the books to you and then return them for you. The library is a great resource for those who have a small child to entertain while on bedrest. The library can put together a reading list for children and possibly recommend activities.

- Stock up on paper plates, plastic forks and spoons, cups, and napkins. These commodities will help a great deal with after dinner clean up for others, as well as your lying in bed wondering how messy your kitchen looks.

- Keep a wastebasket by the bed so you can dispose of items you don't want in your direct living space – napkins, wrappers, paper, and other clutter.

- Keep the "Questions for Doctor Pad" next to the bed so when a question occurs to you, you can write it down. This pad is also great for monitoring contractions and making "honey do lists."

- If you don't already have a babysitter, talk with friends about reliable individuals they use and who can be available to you. Then, schedule times for a sitter to come by, especially if you are on bedrest during the summer months while children are out of school. A sitter who drives can take children to the park, library activities, swimming pool, pick up a few groceries, and run errands.

- If finances permit, hire a lawn care service to maintain your lawn. This will take stress off everyone and allow the family more time together in the evenings and on weekends.

- If finances permit, hire someone to clean your home. This will help everyone feel less stressed and enable your home to stay somewhat presentable. Make a list of items you absolutely want the cleaning person to complete so you feel that your goals have been met. Before having a cleaning person in your home, check references to ensure you and your valuables are safe. A good place to look for a cleaning person is your local church. Often, elderly ladies will take on cleaning jobs to make extra money, and, who knows, maybe your church will help fund this extra expense.

- Keeping yourself occupied during bedrest will be invaluable. The following are some suggested activities for diversion:
  - Read books or listen to audio books.
  - View tapes and/or written materials about childbirth, breastfeeding, and parenting.
  - Listen to sermon tapes from church, if a church attendee.
  - Learn a foreign language – these programs can be obtained from a local library or bookstore.
  - Knit or crochet – this is a great time to make booties, caps and blankets for the future.
  - Needlepoint.
  - Paint – use a lap table to help reduce spills.
  - Write letters to baby, friends, and family.
  - Journal your thoughts, feelings, pregnancy story, etc. Journaling can be in the form of written text, drawings, paintings, etc.
  - Organize recipe cards.
  - Address Christmas cards or other kinds of cards.
  - Address birth announcements.
  - Make a list of things to do when the baby comes.
  - Design the nursery – where to place furniture, what paint and decorations, bedding, etc.
  - Document your pregnancy journey by logging your thoughts, feelings, activities, etc. in a journal daily.
  - Order items for the baby from catalogs and online.
  - Scrapbook.
  - Research child care centers if you will be returning back to work after the baby is born.
  - Organize/assemble photo albums.
  - Email friends and family.
  - Work from home if the profession permits and with your doctor's approval.

o   Help with community activities such as making telephone calls, addressing envelopes for schools, churches and other organizations.
o   Work puzzles, including crossword, word search, and jigsaw puzzles.
o   Play cards – various games with a deck of cards or online with a laptop computer available by the bedside.
o   Learn a new word everyday from the dictionary or online.
o   Play hand held video games – time passes very fast with this activity.
o   Pamper yourself – give yourself a manicure or facial.
o   Mend clothes from the safety of the bed.
o   Fold laundry while sitting up, as permitted by your doctor.
o   Play with your children, keeping your activity limitations in mind.
o   Set up a date night with your partner. You could have an in-bed picnic and movie.
o   Get a professional massage. Check with your doctor before having a massage to ensure it is safe for your pregnancy medical condition. A massage can help with stiff and achy muscles, circulation, and relaxation.
o   Plan meals for your family.
o   Take an online class if your doctor permits.
o   Organize your calendar by denoting special events and occasions.
o   Construct Christmas and birthday gift lists.
o   Baby time – set aside time everyday to close your eyes and feel the physical experience of being pregnant. Remind yourself of how blessed you are to have a little miracle growing inside you. This can be a relaxing and rewarding activity. Goal: keep your mind on the positive aspects of your pregnancy.
o   Support time – set aside time every day or every other day to talk with other mothers experiencing pregnancy bedrest. A list of websites and groups are provided in Appendix A.
o   Go outside a few minutes each day, only if your doctor approves. If you are on hospital bedrest, your doctor may agree to let you be wheeled outside in a wheelchair

for a few minutes to get fresh air and to enjoy a change of scenery.

o Read the newspaper daily. This will help you to feel connected to the outside world and updated on current events. Additionally, it will occupy several hours of time, making the day pass a little faster.

o Listen to music daily. Music is essential for healing the body, mind, and spirit. Devote a portion of each day to listening to your favorite music, either at home or online. The *Pregnancy Relaxation: Body, Mind and Spirit* CD, in the Pregnancy Bedrest Essentials set is excellent for inducing relaxation. The spa sounds sooth the body, mind, and spirit, thereby, reducing anxiety, worry, and restlessness. Additionally, a baby's response to music is amazing. If the music selections are funky and upbeat you may get more kicks and movement, but if the music is sublime you may get more resting and gentle movement. Music sessions are wonderful bonding times. If in the hospital, use headphones so as not to disturb other patients.

o Watch movies during the day. Movies can be ordered online and delivered via US Mail or viewed online. If you do not have a computer, call your local video store and see if they will let you select a movie(s), pay for it by credit card, and mail it to your home or allow someone to pick it up for you. Also, ask friends to share their favorite movies with you. Before long, you will have a large selection of media to choose from. Keep in mind that movies can set your mood. You may want to stay away from sad movies during this time – comedies and lighthearted ones may be best for now.

o Spend time with friends. I can't express how important friends and companions are for bedrest patients. Allow your friends to be there for you; they want to help. Keeping friendships alive during this time will benefit you in ways unimaginable. Also, don't worry about how you look – women know "we all have our less than beauty pageant look moments."

  • Invite friends over for movie night. One lady had her friends come in their pajamas for a slumber party and what a memory they will all cherish.

- Invite friends over for pampering. You can do this by calling your local Mary Kay or other consultants and requesting a makeover party. Most beauty consultants will not pass on the opportunity to create new business, so enjoy your friends, pampering, and the sale's associate possibly attaining new customers.
- Invite friends to your home for coffee, tea, and snacks. Bringing snacks and drinks can be shared by all. This involvement will also allow for down time for the invited persons and for catching up with the girls and sharing a few laughs.
- Have a game night with the girls. Amazingly, many games can be played while lying down. Some fun ones are Scrabble, Taboo, Poker (various card games), and Dominos.
- Let friends help with errands. Make a list of things that need someone's help and ask each friend to volunteer for a week. Friends are valuable for both children and spouses during this time. Friends can help with school activities by providing support at games, and transporting children to and from school and other activities. Friends can provide support by taking the kids a few hours each week or on the weekends, or for evenings so that you and your husband have alone time. Friends can also help with household chores such as cleaning, laundry, and mowing the lawn. Let your friend's help; that's what friends are for.

o Set aside time every day to check in with family to see how everyone is coping with the bedrest situation. Plan fun things such as games, movies, meals, stories, arts, and crafts to do as a family. This time will also allow for reduction in stress and bonding.

o Practice relaxation techniques. Engage in deep breathing and meditation exercises. Finding calm in the midst of a storm is important when dealing with a crisis. Use the relaxation techniques provided in Chapter Six to help reduce stress, anxiety, and muscle tension.

Before long, you will be through this journey and life will return to normal. When all is said and done, you will be able to look back on this phase of your life and know that you did everything you could to help your baby have every chance at life and health – that's being a good mother!

Chapter Four

Parenting Young Children While on Bedrest
Explaining Your Pregnancy Medical Condition
Activity Suggestions for Young Children

᠊ᡟ᠊ᡟ᠊ᡟ᠊ᡟ᠊ᡟ᠊ᡟ᠊ᡟ᠊ᡟ᠊ᡟ᠊ᡟ

Hearing the words "You have to go on bedrest" creates feelings of stress and anxiety for the expectant mother, and if other children are to be cared for during the bedrest time, it can seem an impossible task. "How will I do this and still take care of the children?" is usually the first question that enters the expectant mother's thinking. I remember this initial phase myself. Lydia was two years old when I went on bedrest with Caleb. Thinking of things to entertain myself was difficult enough the first time around. The second time, I also had the task of keeping Lydia entertained and cared for. While caring for Lydia was a challenge, it was not as difficult as I had anticipated. Actually, the days and weeks seemed to pass quicker the second time around and I felt less lonely. Another enjoyable aspect was the quality time she and I spent together during my bedrest. I learned things about her I had never noticed before because of our hectic daily schedules.

If your doctor allows you to provide child care if you have other children while on bedrest, be sure to keep your pregnancy medical condition in mind and not to exceed your physical limitations. Do your best to keep family matters as normal as possible and realize that changes have taken place and adjustments will occur for all affected by the pregnancy bedrest journey. The following is a list of suggestions to help you parent while on bedrest:

- Make sure you keep extra diapers, snacks, drinks, and clothes close by for the child. A small set of stackable plastic drawers is great for storing these items.

44

- Keep all medications and potentially harmful items out of your child's reach.
- Have lots of activities available for entertainment; a list of suggestions is provided at the end of this chapter.
- Make sure your child gets plenty of exercise each day. If your bedrest is strict with only bathroom privileges, have your child be your little helper. This will get him or her up out of the bed and about and don't forget to give praise for your little one's help. Also, after other family members return home in the afternoon and/or evening, encourage outside and inside play that requires physical activity.
- Accept help from family and friends.
- Remember, you are the parent and keep conversation content appropriate. It's easy to lean on your child, especially older children for emotional support but refrain from doing so. Later in this chapter, information pertaining to explaining your medical condition to your children will be provided.
- Set up play dates with friends.
- Look into extended care if your child is school age.
- Sign your child up for activities such as gymnastics, swimming lessons, softball, tee-ball, tennis, etc. If transportation is an issue, get a list of the parents and ask for help with transportation. Make sure you trust the people you are entrusting your children to.
- Provide the school a list of people who will be transporting your child to and from school and include emergency contacts.
- Keep in touch with the teacher and other care givers via email, notes, and telephone conversations to make sure your children are coping and doing what is expected of them.
- Contact your child's pediatrician and inform him/her about your pregnancy condition and find out what documentation will be necessary for them to have on file, should your child need medical attention.
- Make sure you check your child's backpack daily for notes, events, homework assignments, etc.
- Have daily conversations with your children to let them know you are still there for them and a part of their lives. Initiate discussions about school and friends. Ask your child to tell you what was good about the day and what was not so good. This scenario sets the stage for open-ended conversation allowing you to gain insight into what's going on in your child's life outside of the home.

Remember that you are doing the best you can with your situation. Try not to feel guilty about your limited activity level. You will soon be back on your feet running your legs off.

Explaining Your Pregnancy Medical Condition

A parent's lying in bed day after day can be a frightening experience for a child. The child is going from having a mom up and about and being involved in everyday activities to lying in bed experiencing numerous physical limitations. In essence, the child's world has also changed in a moment - just as the mother's who has been prescribed pregnancy bedrest. So, how does the mother stay in bed and keep her child's stress and worry levels low? Personally, I think with planning. Children are observant and will know something less than normal is occurring in the home. Children are little emotional barometers in reference to their parent's emotions. If a parent is having a bad day, too often toddlers will also have a less than "comfortable" day. Intuitively, children take on the primary care givers emotions, thus acting out in the only ways they know how, either positive, negative, and/or in overly needy behaviors. Therefore, it becomes very important to keep young ones in the loop and to keep the loop as normal as possible when dealing with the mother's bedrest issue. Conversation between the parents about behavior expectations are two key factors in accomplishing this goal of maintaining family normalcy.

Children over two years of age will be aware of the changes that come with pregnancy bedrest. They may not be able to articulate their thoughts and feelings well at such a young age, however, they will express them. So, it is important that these young children have something of an understanding about what is going on in the family. A sense of understanding will help them feel safe and loved. For children who are between the ages of two and four years old, stories about life events are an excellent way of getting messages across, as are hands on play with animals, dolls, and toys. Conversation content is also very important. When telling a story, use tone, body language, and content that are positive. Children can read body language and process tone of voice, which, in turn, educates them about how they should be feeling and responding. I will share the story I told Lydia when I found out I was going to have to stay in bed during my second pregnancy:

Once upon a time there was a momma bear who had a beautiful little girl cub with whom she loved to play every day. The momma bear also had another cub, but it was growing in her belly so that it could someday come and play with the little girl cub. One afternoon momma bear said, "I have a little tummy rumbling so I should go see the bear doctor." Momma bear went to see the bear doctor, and he said momma bear was doing okay, but she needed to get a little more rest so that the cub in momma bear's belly could grow big and strong. The bear doctor told momma bear, "Go home, make a soft bed and get little girl cub to help you have fun while you are resting. Tell her to make you laugh, to play in the bed with you, to sing you her favorite songs, and to watch fun shows together." Momma bear thought this was a great idea because she loved spending time with little girl cub. Momma bear went straight home to see little girl cub and shared the good news that they were going to get to play on the bed and spend lots of time together. Little girl cub was happy to get momma bear all to herself and to help the cub in momma bear's belly grow bigger and stronger. The end.

Lydia really took to this story. She asked me to tell it over and over. The content of the story was mild and let Lydia know that while I was going to have to stay in bed, she was still my favorite little girl whom I loved very much. Also, she seemed to feel that she was a part of helping the baby grow and come safely into the world. At Lydia's age, I chose not to get detailed about medical issues because I did not want to create worry in her heart and mind, and she could not comprehend information about a medical condition at the age of two. The body language I displayed when Lydia and I were together was one of excitement. By telling her she needed to play with me, sing songs, and help me have fun, made her feel like a big girl. Inside, I was struggling with concerns, fear, sadness, and a lot of other emotions; however, my job was to parent both of my children the best I knew how; so, I did – just as you will.

Be aware that children four years old and up will ask more questions and want to know specifics. Again, keep your conversation content appropriate. For a child who is four you might say something similar to the following:

Your little baby brother/sister in my belly is trying to come out and play a little too soon, so the doctor wants me to rest and keep him/her inside as long as I can so that your brother/sister can grow nice and big like you. I will not be able to do all of the things we usually do, but I have a bunch of great things we can do while I lie in bed. We can read stories together, watch our favorite movies

47

*while eating popcorn, draw pictures, sing songs, and my favorite –
laugh. I can't wait for all us to spend time together. I love you
and will always be here for you.*

For a child who is seven or eight (depending on their maturity level),
you may want to be a little more content specific about your bedrest
situation. However, avoid being overly detailed about medical issues, as
this can create worry and fear in the heart and mind of a small child. Make
sure the child knows you are handling everything and that he or she has
nothing to worry about. By this age, the child will be able to help around
the house, so encourage participation in cleaning, laundry, and other
chores. Be sure to show your appreciation and point out how special you
feel because they care so much about you, the baby, and family.

For older children, let them know what is going on, but spare them the
intense details, and, above all, do not use them as your emotional sounding
board. Your children love you and do not want to see you suffer, and, if
you explicitly share your suffering with them, they will take on your
emotional burdens. You may feel better after unloading, but they are going
to feel worse. This is not to say "lie" to them, but let them know that your
bedrest condition is not an easy task for you to accomplish, but that you
want to do what is necessary because you love the baby growing inside of
you just as you love them. Remind your children that you would do the
same thing for them and that families sacrifice for each other. Encourage a
spirit of helpfulness and giving during this time, and help the whole family
embark on this journey as a team who wants to support each other.
Explain you are still there for your children and will do all you can to stay
involved in their lives, but that they have to take some responsibility in
keeping you in the loop by helping you stay up to date on what's going on
in their lives outside of the home.

You will be amazed at how well your children will respond to your
pregnancy bedrest situation if you handle it with positive framing.
Children are resilient; they adapt to change quite well if given time. Try to
keep a positive outlook during this trying time of life. You will have days
when you don't feel positive and that's okay. Just try to limit those days
and remember not to unload or take out your stress on your children who
are also going through changes. It's okay to say, "Mommy needs to be
alone for a little while to rest and think." You will be modeling positive
self-expression and the ability to ask for what you need. Before long this
journey will be complete and you will be back in the thick of family life
once again.

Websites and Activity Suggestions

I am hopeful that the following websites and activity suggestions will be helpful to mothers on bedrest in keeping small ones entertained.

Websites:
- Coloring pages can be printed from these various websites:
  www.PBSkids.org
  www.NickJr.com
  www.PlayhouseDisney.com
  www.PollyPocket.com

- The following websites are good sites for story time:
  www.Mightybook.com
  www.lil-fingers.com
  www.PBSKids.org

- Online Games
  www.Meddybemps.com
  www.Boowakwala.com
  www.PBSkids.org
  www.NickJr.com
  www.PlayhouseDisney.com
  www.PollyPocket.com
  www.Barbie.com

Activity Suggestions:
- Design Cup Dolls:
  Assimilate plastic cups, fabric, buttons, glitter, glue, yarn, sequins, etc. Glue the supplies on to the cup to make faces and hair. If you do not have scraps of fabric, use an old shirt or towel and cut them into shapes.

- Clothes Pin People:
  Take a clothes pin and glue a cotton ball on top for hair and use markers to draw faces and clothes.

- Hair Salon:
  Pretend to need a new hair style and ask your little one to give you a make-over. This is fun for both since having your hair brushed (gently) is relaxing. Your child can pretend to cut your hair with

his/her fingers and add hair clips and bows. This is a great picture moment!

- In-Bed Picnic:
  Spread a table cloth on the bed and eat lunch together while lying on one side. Let your child serve you and enjoy creativity. Tell stories about your favorite days and/or events from childhood.

- Bed Basketball:
  Place a small wastebasket at the foot of the bed. Wad up pieces of paper and try throwing them into the wastebasket. Each successful basket can earn a letter to spell a word, such as cat, dog, pig, horse, love, etc. Again, while lying on one side.

- Play Dough or Clay Shapes:
  Have your child make special sculptures with play dough or clay. Let each creation dry, then paint and decorate with glitter, buttons, etc.

- Draw on a Mirror with Dry-Erase Markers:
  Hold the mirror and let your child draw silly faces. It's "cute" for the child to look at you and try to draw your face. They are very creative.

- Create Shape Puzzles:
  Foamies are great for this project. However, other materials, such as cardboard, paper, fabric, rubber, and foam can be used. Draw designs/shapes on chosen product and have the child color with crayons/markers/chalk. Cut out the shapes and let your child re-assemble the pieces to complete the puzzle.

- Binoculars:
  Take two empty toilet paper rolls and glue them together to resemble binoculars. If the eye pieces are too close together for your child, try gluing something, such as a small piece of sponge or a cotton ball between the two rolls. Use the binoculars to explore the room.

- Dry Food Collage:
  Using a paper plate, a piece of cardboard, or poster paper, let your child glue items such as pasta, cereal, beans, candy, etc. to create a collage.

- Mommy and Me Collage:
  Using a paper plate, a piece of cardboard, or poster paper, let your child glue photos of the two of you onto the product to create a collage.

- Sewing Cards:
  Glue a page from a coloring book onto a piece of cardboard. Allow your child to color and then punch holes around the edge of the design. Give your child a shoe string to lace through the holes.

- Personal Puppet:
  Cut out photos of child and family members and glue them onto popsicle sticks, then have a puppet show with funny voices.

- Eye Spy:
  Play a game of eye spy with items or colors. "Eye spy with my little eye something the color of ...."

- Popcorn Jewelry:
  Pop some popcorn and string it onto thread. This activity can also be done with buttons, beads, cereal, etc. These creations make great necklaces and bracelets.

- Me Masks:
  Use a paper plate and cut out two circles for the eyes and color or paint the plate for skin tone. Use construction paper and cut out and paste on a mouth, ears, nose and eyebrows. Glue on yarn for hair. Make the mask look like your child. Have your child make one that looks like you and pretend to be at a masquerade party and guess who is behind the mask.

- Sock Puppets:
  Take an old pair of socks and draw, paint or glue eyes, nose, and mouth onto the socks. Place the socks over the child's hand and make the puppets move and talk.

- Hanger People:
  Take a hanger and cover it with plain white paper or use a white paper hanger from the dry cleaners. Take a small paper plate, and, using crayons, markers, and/or paint, make a child's face. Using a piece of tape, glue the plate near the top of the hanger hook. Next, use a sheet of paper to trace around your child's hands and feet. Glue or tape the hands and feet onto the hanger. When you finish, you have your very own hanger person that represents your child.

- Paper Butterflies:
  Provide a piece of paper and let your child color it with crayons or markers. Fold the piece of paper accordion style (back and forth) in inch wide sections. Take a pipe cleaner and wrap it around the middle of the paper, giving a couple of twists to secure it. Let your child bend or twist the excess pipe cleaner stems to make butterfly antennae.

- Riddle, Riddle, Marie:
  Say "Riddle, riddle, Marie, I see something you don't see and the color of it is...." The child then guesses what object has the correct color.

- Rock Collection:
  For a child who is past putting things in his/her mouth, collecting rocks is a lot of fun. Your child can collect rocks and bring them back inside to be examined by a magnifying glass. This can also be done with leaves and sticks.

- Popsicle Stick Construction:
  Glue popsicle sticks together to create a house, triangle, etc.

- Mommy and Me Journal:
  Take a blank notebook and invite your child to write stories and draw pictures of your times together.

- Write letters:
  Encourage your child who knows how to read and write to write letters to family and friends.

- Write books:
  Have your child tell you a story and then you write the words and sketch the pictures about the story; your child will not care about your drawing abilities. This will be a fun activity to reflect on even after the bedrest journey has ended.

- Play School:
  Get a small chalk board/dry erase board and practice letters, numbers, spelling, math, and other academic skills. Take turns being the teacher.

- Movie Date:
  Allow your child to pick out a movie for the both of you to view. If popcorn is on your diet, enjoy it with your child during the move.

- Board Games:
  Play games such as Monopoly, Yahtzee, Candyland, Bingo, and any other game that your child enjoys.

- Read Stories:
  Get a basket/backpack of books together and read a least one story per day to your children. Additionally, have a story hour every week and wear a funny hat while reading - kids love this.

- Outside Play:
  If your doctor approves your being outside, take a cot outside or lie on a lounge chair and watch your child play. This is a great time to play "Eye Spy" with your child.

Chapter Five

Common Emotions Experienced and Suggestions for Emotional Relief

❖❖❖❖❖❖❖❖❖❖❖

When faced with the challenge of pregnancy bedrest, a woman can, and often does, experience a gamut of emotions – some positive, some negative, some in between. Think about it, you are going along with life: working, engaged in home and family activities, and being socially involved, then, suddenly, you are told "Go to bed." One minute you are up and out in the world, and what seems to be the next minute you are confined to the house or hospital. Your plans have changed and, likely, very suddenly. Along with these changes in activity, emotional changes will surface as well.

The goal I hope to meet in this chapter is providing a sense of permission to be who you are at this particular time in your life. Also, I hope to provide some coping strategies that will help you get through what may seem an endless journey. Everyone copes with life stressors differently, so accepting your present situation and making conscious decisions about how you will manage your pregnancy bedrest journey is an important decision. While it may feel there are no positive things going on in your life because of the drastic changes that come with bedrest, if you dig deep enough you will find many positives. My challenge to you is to look at your life situation with hope instead of despair and turn your bedrest obstacles into opportunities.. The following is a list of stages, emotions, and thoughts you may experience while enduring bedrest:

- *Denial*: Denial is an unconscious self-defense mechanism which allows for avoiding thoughts, feelings, and realities that bring about emotional discomfort and pain. An example of denial that comes to mind is one from my first complicated pregnancy experience. My doctor encouraged me to visit the neonatal intensive care unit (NICU) so I could educate myself about preterm babies just in case my baby was born with physical complications. Each time I went to the hospital I avoided the NICU. I refused to believe my baby might need assistance to survive. I told myself, "It's not going to happen, so why put myself through the trauma." The truth is I could not handle seeing those little babies hooked up to all the medical equipment. I avoided the pain that could come with accepting this reality.

While denial is a common emotion often experienced when faced with a crisis, it is important to work beyond this emotion. Had my daughter been born with complications, she would have been placed in the NICU and I would have been ignorant to what took place because of my own denial to her situation. Accepting life circumstances that bring about emotional pain can take time. Give yourself time, and realize you have immeasurable strength when put to the test. Facing the fear that comes with difficult truths is a challenge and an opportunity to prepare for the future. To overcome those fears, educate yourself about your condition and talk with others who have been in your situation. Hearing positive stories can bring hope, which, in turn, brings strength to face fear. If I had accepted the fact my baby would possibly need assistance from the NICU, I would have educated myself and learned that many preterm babies do very well and only need minimal assistance. I would have been able to let go of some of the secret fears I kept hidden in my heart and mind for months.

- *Anger:* Anger can be described as having intense feelings of displeasure. Having dreams of a healthy, normal pregnancy shattered can bring about feelings of anger and disappointment. "Why me?" is a question all pregnancy bedrest patients likely entertain; I know I certainly did. "Why is my body doing this to me?" "Why can't my doctor make this better – he/she is considered a healer?" "Why do I have to leave work?" The list could go on and on. When posing such questions, the goal is to make sense out of an otherwise senseless situation. The down side is that you may never get the answers to the questions, and that lack of closure can bring about feelings of loss of control over life. A feeling of having no control over a life's situation can also create feelings of anger.

55

Experiencing feelings of anger is a normal part of life. Being in touch with how to feel in relation to life changes that are not pleasant or desired is what striving for functional mental health is about. Once a move from denial is made, the individual will likely feel angry, which is a part of the healing process. However, it is important to keep in mind that anger can have both positive and negative aspects. Anger that motivates looking inside oneself and seeking change and direction is positive. Anger directed inward that brings shame and self-devaluation is negative. Also, anger that is projected onto others with an unconscious or conscious attempt to inflict pain (emotional or physical) is not the appropriate way to handle feelings. So, it's important to assess where, as a bedrest patient, you are and what you are feeling and to make decisions based on where you want to be.

Again, remember, it's okay to feel anger during this demanding life situation; who wouldn't when faced with a complicated pregnancy, especially one that requires bedrest for many weeks. But, try not to get stuck in the anger stage. The following is a list of ways to help direct in processing feelings of anger and find healing.

- o Acknowledge your feelings of anger and disappointment. Know that all persons feel angry and disappointed at times, especially when things don't work out as planned. Anger, of itself, is just an emotion. The significant aspect of anger is deciding what to do with it and deciding at what level you will allow your anger to control aspects of your life.
- o Assess your emotions and determine if anger is justified, and it may be. If so, remember harboring feelings of anger hurts only you in the long run. Determine if forgiveness is an option and know that we all deserve to heal and move on.
- o Come to understand the stem of anger: a pregnancy situation, anger at someone in your life, anger with yourself, or other factors.
- o Work on accepting your current life situations and know you are not being punished. Sometimes the body does what the body wants to do and little control is to be had.

- Address the feelings of loss of control. Know that you are not completely out of control. While you cannot control how your body is responding to pregnancy, you do have control over how you respond to your pregnancy and other events taking place in your life.
- Journal your feelings daily. This will allow you to process your thoughts and feelings without the fear of judgment from others and will allow you to externalize your feelings, which will bring a sense of relief.
- Talk to others, either partner, family, friends, doctor, therapist and/or clergy about your feelings. Ask for advice on processing anger in a healthy manner.
- Think about the behaviors and thoughts that trigger your feelings of anger and come to understand where these emotions are rooted. Work on becoming less reactive to negative stimuli.
- Create a list of things that sooth and calm you, keeping your pregnancy situation in mind. Implement these strategies when feeling angry or frustrated.
- Take a deep breath when becoming angry and count to ten, and then exhale. Give yourself time to turn your anger down a few notches before responding. Practice relaxation exercises described in Chapter Six.
- If you have small children, work it out that you have some time to yourself everyday. Stress and anxiety can run high for the mother on bedrest. (You don't want to have to deal with the guilt of projecting your anger on your children, nor do they deserve it.)
- Remember, there will be time for work in the future, if you are experiencing feelings of anger about having to leave a job that you truly enjoy. However, your baby has only a short period of time for growth. Priorities are a must at this stage in the game. You have the most important job in the world right now – bringing a baby into it.

- *Guilt*: Guilt can be defined as feeling as if your actions have affected others and yourself negatively; in other words, a sense of loss. "Did I do something to cause my pregnancy complications?" I'm sure every woman experiencing a difficult pregnancy has asked that question. It's human nature to need understanding; that's why we question. During my first preterm labor experience,

I remember asking my doctor over and over "Are you sure I didn't cause this to happen?" I was consumed with guilt, even though I knew in my mind that I had done everything I should have done to have a healthy pregnancy.

In addition to the guilt associated with a less than normal pregnancy, guilt can also arise from feeling you are not carrying your weight in the family as you normally did. I could present a list of things a woman might feel guilty about when placed on pregnancy bedrest, but I prefer not to do that. I don't want to be the supplier of the stick you use to beat-up yourself – I'm sure you likely have a comprehensive list already. However, I will say, you are doing the best you can in a difficult situation. While others may have to take on household duties they are not accustomed to performing, experiencing financial changes, enduring lack of physical intimacy with your partner, and other adversities know that you are doing what is best for you, your baby and family, and that the situation has to be good enough for now.

No guilt should be involved in loving your unborn child. He or she is counting on you for survival. Don't allow yourself to disregard your doctor's orders because of feeling guilty about things going on around you. When the pregnancy bedrest journey ends, there will be laundry to do, meals to cook, the house to clean, and, for some, a job to return to outside of the home. You may even find yourself in the future longing for a few days of down time to get a break. The following ideas may help alleviate feelings of guilt:

- o The majority of pregnancy complications come about as a result of the body's response to pregnancy. Try not to get caught up in the blame game. If you are unable to convince yourself you did nothing to bring on your medical condition, talk with your doctor. He or she will be able to give you facts to alleviate the feeling of being responsible. If, by chance, some behavior you or someone else in your life displayed brought about your pregnancy complications, take responsibility and offer yourself forgiveness and vow to learn from your mistakes and move on. Beating yourself up will not make your situation better.

o Talk with your partner about your feelings of guilt. I am most confident the response to that endeavor will be, "You have nothing to feel guilty about and you have the most important job in the world right now just taking care of our baby."

o Talk with other women on pregnancy bedrest about your feelings of guilt and don't be surprised when they express the exact same feelings.

o Journal your feelings. Externalizing your thoughts helps to lessen the load.

o Nurture yourself by pointing out all you have done right during your pregnancy and all you are willing to contribute to helping your baby.

o When thinking you are lazy because you lie in bed all day, remember you would give your right arm to be playing with your other children if you have other children or working, gardening, shopping, and socializing. You are not in bed because of laziness, but because of strong commitment to getting the present job done.

o If you have other children in the household and are experiencing guilt about not being as active with those children, address the issue head on. Explain the significance of what you are doing and how you would do the same for your other children if they needed you to do so. Also, be sure to keep the content of your conversations in relation to your medical and emotional condition age appropriate. Being too explicit to your children can create fear and stress – they don't need it nor do you. Remind them you are a family and families sacrifice for each other. Include them in the journey so they don't feel left out and you don't feel the guilt of separation.

• *Anxiety and Fear*: Anxiety and fear seem to go hand in hand for any woman experiencing a complicated pregnancy. Keeping in mind that anxiety is a normal part of life for all of us is important to remember. A Chinese proverb, "A little anxiety helps to focus the mind, but too much paralyzes it" is significant for the bedrest mother to remember. Anxiety can be both positive and negative and differentiating between the two becomes the goal. An example of positive anxiety for the bedrest mother is mild worry brought about by the possibility of forgetting to take prescribed medication in the middle of the night; therefore, she would set the alarm clock in order not to miss a dose and to recheck it a few times before drifting off to sleep. Negative anxiety could be worrying so much about forgetting to take prescribed medication that the bedrest mother becomes unable to fall asleep, even after setting the alarm out of fear of not waking up on time. One type of anxiety motivates the other debilitates.

Anxiety is both a psychological and physiological experience. The psychological aspects of anxiety are worried thoughts, inability to concentrate, focusing on the worse possible outcome, irritability, mood swings, and overwhelming fear. The physical aspects of anxiety tend to be a racing heart, increased rate of breathing, nausea or stomach pain, tension in muscles, headaches, dizziness, excessive crying, and decrease/increase in appetite. Keep in mind, however, some medications prescribed for complicated pregnancies have side effects similar to symptoms associated with anxiety. Yet, the difference between chemically induced anxiety and psychologically induced anxiety can usually be discerned. If the cause of anxiety is questionable, speak with your doctor and he or she will be able to help you weed out the cause.

Becoming anxious when big changes take place in life is normal. Going from what seems a normal pregnancy to sudden bedrest is a huge change. While some level of anxiety is normal, it's also important to understand when anxiety has passed the bounds of normality. The expectant mother having some worries about her unborn baby is not abnormal; mothers are wired this way. However, if the worry about a bedrest pregnancy is having a negative impact on life, including not eating, not sleeping, experiencing constant fear, panic attacks, or other complications then the anxiety needs to be addressed by a professional.

The following is a list of symptoms exemplary of anxiety:

o Excessive worrying.
o Excessive crying.
o Avoidance and withdrawal behavior.
o Sleeping difficulties ranging from more than just a few times and not medication induced.
o Reduction in appetite.

60

- Weight loss or excessive weight gain not appropriate to pregnancy bedrest.
- Inappropriate display/internalization of anger.
- Excessive irritability.
- Negative outlook.
- Increased heart rate – feeling panicked.
- Shortness of breath.
- Sweaty hands.
- Inability to concentrate.
- Intense muscle pain and tension.

If your anxiety level is not normal for your life situation, then please talk with your doctor, a mental health therapist, partner, family, friends, clergy, or someone else who can offer professional advice.

Tips for managing anxiety:

- Eat a well balanced diet and reduce sugar intake.
- Eliminate caffeine from your diet.
- Get necessary rest.
- Establish routines, including certain time for meals, showering, telephone calls, sleeping, etc. Keep in mind not to let a routine become a stressor, but a stress reducer. Try to be flexible.
- Create a nightly routine before going to bed which allows gradual relaxation: read a book, drink warm milk and/or eat a snack, listen to relaxation music, perform meditation, etc.
- Make a list of worries and put them in a container. Allow yourself time to look at the list every day, then put the list away with the thought "Worry time is over for today; I can do it again tomorrow if I need to." This exercise actually does work if a commitment is made to it.
- Practice letting go by remembering you can't control every aspect of your life, the house, yard, health, and children. Work on accepting what you can control and how you approach your life stressors.
- Determine the negative self-talk creating your anxiety and focus on putting a more positive spin on these thoughts through the process of reframing.

o Mental imagery relaxation – close your eyes and visualize relaxing places and things. Allow yourself the opportunity to escape from bedrest into this relaxing image created in your mind.

o Positive thinking – think of how you can look at life through positive lenses instead of negative ones.

o Relaxation music – listen to relaxation music and allow your body, mind, and spirit to calm.

o Bedrest physical exercises – only ones approved by your doctor.

o Find pleasurable things to keep your mind off your worries. Idle time is the great precursor for anxiety and, when on bedrest, you have plenty of time. So try and keep yourself occupied.

Some of the items listed above will be discussed in greater detail in Chapter Six that includes positive thinking, deep breathing, muscle relaxation, and guided-imagery exercises. You may have to practice learning to relax and letting go of negative, controlling thoughts, but you can do it. Bedrest is a perfect time for honing these skills. They will be a great asset for your upcoming years of parenting.

- *Grief*: The feeling of grief comes from losing something or someone who is important. The emotions surrounding grief can range from mild to intense, depending on the interpretation of the extent of loss. The French describe the state of bereavement as having been robbed. I like this interpretation from the standpoint of a woman facing a complicated pregnancy. Many women experiencing bedrest do feel robbed. I recall thinking, "I have worked very hard at being good, at being pregnant, and now I feel that the positive aspects of my pregnancy have been stolen from me." Women have a plan in their mind about pregnancy (especially the first time around), and when things don't work out as planned, we end up feeling a sense of loss. The loss is real – not just perceived. Depending on the strictness of the pregnancy bedrest prescription, there can be loss of work, income, and control over the body along with a decrease in health, dreams, and hopes.

Remember, time is the healer of all wounds so give yourself time and permission to grieve your losses. Before you know it, you will be back on your feet living life with your precious gift in tow. The following is a list of tips for managing grief:

- Allow yourself time. Every person's response to loss is different; therefore, the grieving time varies from person to person. However, the sooner you are able to accept changes and losses, the sooner your grieving process will become less.
- Educate yourself about the grieving process. This will help you understand what to expect.
- Connect with supportive and caring people. Establish a network of friends, family, and other bedrest women who offer positive support and suggestions. Sharing stories about life struggles with others and how to overcome those struggles can create bonds and offer healing. The volunteers with Sidelines.org (a national non-profit organization offering support to women on bedrest) are very helpful for the expectant mother and family during this life challenge.
- Work on accepting the changes that have taken place in your life. Acknowledge there are things in life beyond your control, and choose to move forward rather than focusing on the past.
- Ask for help. Let others know what you need from them to help you get through this time of grieving.
- Monitor your emotions – especially your anger. It's not uncommon for anger to be displayed when people are dealing with grief. Sometimes it is difficult to be vulnerable enough to express your feelings (hurt, sadness, or loneliness) in relation to loss, so anger emerges.
- Talk with your doctor about symptoms of grief, symptoms such as sleeplessness, change in eating habits, and/or hopelessness.
- Nurture yourself. Remind yourself you are a good mother and you are doing everything possible to help keep your unborn baby safe.
- Remind yourself you are a strong woman who has overcome life's struggles in the past and that you will do the same this time.

- *Isolation and loneliness*: Feeling isolated and lonely is characterized by a sense of abandonment and/or disconnected from others. This feeling of isolation can be real or perceived. Real in the sense you may have to spend a great deal of time alone because of a working partner, children at school all day, not being able to work or interact with others on a daily basis, or no shopping. Perceived in that you may feel you are the only person in the world experiencing the stress of pregnancy bedrest.

Feeling isolated and lonely are common feelings for a woman on bedrest because of much alone time. While being able to alleviate these feelings completely may be difficult, I hope the following tips will help in managing them.

  o Read a newspaper every day – this will help to update you on current events and may present conversation topics with family and friends.
  o Watch the local television news daily.
  o Contact local churches and women's groups to find volunteers in the community that visit shut-ins.
  o Invite friends over for coffee, cards, manicure/pedicure parties, or just girl time.
  o If you have other children, stay in touch with their teachers for updates on how the children are doing in school. This contact can be accomplished via email, telephone, or backpack, among other ways.
  o Check with the library for mobile book groups.
  o If you have a pastor, ask him or her to send weekly service tapes, so you know what is happening at church and with the parishioners in your church.
  o Write letters and/or emails to friends. Receiving responses will provide the sense of connection you are use to when things are normal.
  o Write letters to your unborn baby.
  o If you have other children, write letters to them during the day while they are away at school. When they get home you can review your day, letting them know you were thinking about them and continuing the closeness between you. Also, it will facilitate conversation about their day allowing you to stay in the loop of what is going on outside of the home.

o   Keep in touch with people from work. Follow your doctor's orders if you are allowed to continue working from home, but don't over do it or bring more stress into your life. You have an important job at home to accomplish just keeping you and your baby safe.

o   Schedule time with your children each day, this is important for them as well as yourself. Your kids may be grieving the loss of your being active. Give them permission to talk about their feelings to help with feeling more connected and less lonely for all involved.

o   If you have a pet, allow yourself to enjoy the love and affection a pet can offer.

o   Schedule time with your mate daily to check on how he is coping and report how you are feeling. While it's easy to get self absorbed and focus only on yourself, remember your situation affects others too.

o   Talk about feeling lonely and/or isolated. Getting reassurance from others that they are there for you helps significantly.

o   Talk and read to your baby. Knowing you have a little life growing inside of you is proof that you are not alone on this journey. He or she is cheering you on for success.

- *Loss of Control*: Feeling as if you have to sit on the sidelines and watch the world continue as before without a great deal of participation from you can make a woman feel as if she has lost control over her life. Please know this is a very common feeling for a woman experiencing bedrest. The number one question becomes "How do I take back some control from a situation that seems out of control?" The following are some suggestion to ease the stress:

  o   Think of things in your life that have stayed constant during this stressful time. If you have difficulty coming up with the constants in your life, ask your partner to help you make a list.

  o   Think about your pregnancy situation and what the consequences might be if you do not follow the doctor's orders. You do have a choice to following his/her advice. This decision is control. Of course, you make the decision to follow the doctor's orders because you have the health of your unborn baby as a priority.

- o You have control over the things you say in your head (self-talk). Self-talk can be negative or positive. If you chose to make it negative, you will find yourself wallowing in your difficult pregnancy, but if you choose to make the best out of a difficult situation, focusing on positive self-talk, you will feel stronger and find strength and growth from this experience. This isn't to say you will never have a bad day; however, you have some control over how many bad days you will experience.

- o Stay focused on the prize. Think about people who endure physical and emotional stress to reach a set goal. They have to stay focused on what is to come rather than focusing on their current misery; that's your goal, staying focused on the end result as opposed to the daily stresses of bedrest.

- o Plan your days and make them full without bringing undue stress to your life. If you have other children, you can help them with their homework, plan meals, provide shopping lists, select movies for family movie night, call shut-ins from your church if you belong to a church, and be in contact with other community organizations of which you might be a member. You are still very much a part of everything going on, you just have to be creative and find new ways of continuing your involvement. For example, a lady who was experiencing hospital bedrest had her teenage son ride the school bus to the hospital every day after school. She and her son would have snack time and homework time while waiting for her husband to get off work. She reported amazing conversations between her and her son - it was a special bonding time for the two of them.

- o Remind yourself everyday "My journey of bedrest is going to end someday; it's not forever." It may feel it is at times; however, your participation in this most important journey is of immeasurable value. You are choosing your baby's life! The purest example of a mother's love is her willingness to give the best she has to give.

- *Depression*: Numerous classifications of depression exist on which I could focus; however, after researching depression in relation to women experiencing pregnancy bedrest, it seems that addressing situational depression might be the topic of most benefit. Situational depression is experiencing depressive symptoms as a result of a difficult life situation(s). While the symptoms of situational depression are similar to other depressive disorders, these symptoms tend to be alleviated when life changes start moving again toward the positive realm. I will state, however, that if you have a clinical diagnosis or history in relation to situational or any other type of depression, be sure to keep in touch with your doctor. Unfortunately, even normal pregnancy conditions can bring about depression in some women, and bedrest can complicate this issue more.

The following is list of situational depression symptoms a bedrest mother may experience:

- o Change in emotions such as denial, guilt, or anger.
- o Change in mood such as irritability, nervousness, or anxiousness.
- o Change in social responses such as withdrawal, isolation, arguing, and, perhaps, negative interactions with people/situations you normally enjoy.
- o Decrease in concentration levels (more than normal for pregnancy bedrest patients).
- o Extreme sadness and/or crying.
- o Obsessive thoughts of the traumatic event.
- o Changes in sleeping and eating habits; recurrent nightmares are also a possibility.
- o Thoughts of harming yourself or others.

Although a women prescribed bedrest may not experience all of the symptoms listed, it is likely she will experience some of them. Does this mean all bedrest mother's will experience depression? Not necessarily. However, it would be a good idea to be aware of behavioral changes just in case they do become an issue that needs to be addressed while on bedrest.

Being aware of your feelings and daily responses to your feelings are important if you want to get through bedrest as unscathed as

67

possible. While you have to stay in bed for the safety of your baby, and possibly yourself, that does not mean you have to be miserable. If you struggle with symptoms of situational depression, talk to your doctor. He or she understands bedrest can be a difficult task for women. Many insurance companies will pay for a mental health provider to come to your home or hospital room to provide treatment, if needed. However, you may have to ask for the care. In addition to your doctor and mental health care provider, other areas of support can be your partner, clergy, friends, and online support groups.

Admitting to yourself that you might be experiencing depression can be difficult. However, asking for help is a sign of courage, not cowardice. Acknowledging you are struggling emotionally and choosing to accept the stage you are in is the first step to finding the healing you so deserve. One of my personal struggles while on bedrest was being open with my feelings of situational depression. "I'm a therapist; I should be able to avoid the pitfalls of depression" were the thoughts that went through my mind. I didn't want others to perceive me as weak and unable to practice what I daily preach. Therefore, I suppressed my feelings, hoping those emotions would just go away. One afternoon I was having a telephone conversation with a friend who is also a member of the mental health profession. She asked "How are you doing emotionally with all of this?" My response was, "I'm fine – I can do it." Her response was, "You don't have to put up a strong front; I'm here for you and I want to be here for you." At first, I felt somewhat offended "How dare she challenge me about my feelings and my emotional health." She didn't know what was going on inside my mind and heart.

The more I thought about her comments, the more I realized she was trying to support me and that I was in denial! We had known each other for many years and shared many feelings. She knew I was struggling and was attempting to offer permission for me to be who I was at that moment in time; a normal human being. As a woman, a two-time bedrest patient, and a mental health professional, I want to offer the same advice to you, "be just who you are." Take care of yourself emotionally as well as physically! Holding in your emotions and letting them fester will only cause you more pain and distress. Additionally, these feelings may overlap into the postpartum period if not managed during the bedrest period, thus making recovery more complicated. The following is a good list of self-help strategies if you are struggling with situational depression:

o   Give yourself permission to grieve and experience your feelings.
o   Talk with friends, family members, clergy, mental health professional, doctor, and others about your feelings. Don't be afraid to ask for support from the people in your life. Again, remember they want to help you.
o   Limit your conversations about the situation which is making you feel depressed. This is not to recommend denial, but rather to focus on conversations that bring positive feelings for you.
o   Consider finding a support-group. There are numerous online pregnancy bedrest support groups. These women are in the same boat as you. Just remember not to focus solely on the negative aspects, but to focus also on the positive things occurring in your life.
o   Develop a daily routine.
o   Keep a mood log so you can monitor your fluctuations. This will allow you to pinpoint some of the triggers and help you assess your level of depression.
o   Speak with your doctor about a physical therapy routine while on bedrest. Exercise can help bring about feelings of control over your body and environment. Exercise is also important to mental health wellbeing. <u>You must get your doctors permission first</u>!
o   Think about the things you say to yourself in your mind. Determine if you are making yourself depressed with negative thoughts. If this is happening, work on turning negative thoughts into more positive, less debilitating thoughts.
o   Avoid becoming depressed about your depression. Ask for help; you deserve peace and happiness.
o   Read self-help books on overcoming depression.
o   Continue using any approved medication for depression and/or anxiety prescribed by your doctor and/or OB/GYN. If you feel the medications are not making a difference, don't just stop taking them because doing so can be a

danger with some antidepressants. Talk with your doctor and the two of you can develop a plan of action.

o Remember the serenity prayer: "God, grant me the serenity to accept the things I cannot change, courage to change the things I can, and wisdom to know the difference."

While some women will not battle depression while on pregnancy bedrest, others will. If you are struggling with symptoms of situational depression or other depressive issues, talk with your doctor or seek out other means of support. Should thoughts of self-harm or suicide come about, contact a health care provider, a family member, or trusted friend immediately for help. The National Hopeline Network is (800) 784-2433 for crisis counseling and 911 is also an option. The goal of pregnancy bedrest is to take care of you and your baby, so hang in there!

Chapter Six

Benefits of Relaxation
Relaxation Techniques
Positive Thinking

༄ ༄ ༄ ༄ ༄ ༄ ༄ ༄ ༄ ༄

When reflecting on my pre-pregnancy years, I don't recall experiencing stress or anxiety when thinking about having a baby. What I recall was a strong desire to be a mother and the excitement about what motherhood would hold for me. The thrill that came with learning I was pregnant was wonderful, and, yet, it wasn't long before feelings of worry and anxiety began to creep into my thinking. I recall "what if" questions even before the pregnancy bedrest journey began. Maybe it's human nature to wonder and worry about the unknown. Maybe, for some of us, worry and anxiety are just part of how we respond to life changes. Whatever the reason, many women today are being robbed of the joy of pregnancy. With work, family, social activities, pregnancy medical complications, and demands from other aspects of life, a great number of women are unable to sit back, close their eyes, take a deep breath and connect with the little person growing inside of them. We have to fit in moments for contemplation here and there, and a lot of times we find ourselves unable to relax when we do have the time.

The goal of this chapter is to remind women that while nine months may feel like a long time, especially if several of those months are spent in bed, in the scheme of things it's a very short period. Learning to take one day at a time and live in that day is a gift so many pregnant women need. The hope is that the information presented in this chapter will help you focus on the benefits of relaxation and techniques to accomplish the goal of relaxation. Remember, there is a miracle growing inside of you so experience all that you can; this time can never be reclaimed. You may have another pregnancy, but each is individual to the unborn child.

71

Benefits of Relaxation

Learning to relax allows the body to take a break from the physical, emotional, and mental stresses of day-to-day pressures. By allowing both the mind and body to relax, you will learn to unwind and bring muscle tension and anxiety under control. Relaxation benefits the body in the following ways:

- Reduces fatigue: The body uses more energy to keep muscles tense than to keep them relaxed. Not only does the body use more energy when tense, it also uses more energy when feeling worried or anxious. Persons with anxiety experience an increase in heart rate which brings about rapid breathing, thereby, requiring more oxygen use and an elevation in blood pressure, as well as increased muscle tension. Learning to relax will allow you to conserve more energy and feel calmer, as well as provide better means of coping with your pregnancy situation.
- Reduces pain: When the body becomes tense, common side effects are headaches, backaches, and neck pain. Practicing muscle relaxation exercises can help reduce pain as well as coping with pain by raising the pain threshold. Lying in bed for weeks on end in the same basic position makes the body stiff and the muscles tense. Learning to relax your muscles will help provide relief from the physical pain endured by the pregnancy bedrest patient.
- Reduces anxiety and worry: Pregnancy bedrest will bring worry and anxiety for the expectant parents. Learning to relax and turn down or turn off the "head talk" that creates anxiety and worry is a gift. By relaxing your body, mind, and spirit you will allow healing to take place in life and make this challenging time less challenging. Calming the mind and body will help resolve difficulties relating to sleep, eating, depression, grief, anger, and other adverse emotions and will help to maintain and/or to restore a sense of joy about your pregnancy.

Relaxation Techniques

Prior to starting relaxation exercises, empty your bladder, dim the lights to a comfortable non-intrusive level, reduce all external noises as low as possible, and focus only on yourself. Be mindful of your breathing to keep it slow and not to tighten your abdominal muscles. All of the following exercises can be performed with or without music. Keep in mind, learning to relax is an art - you may need a little practice, so don't give up if it doesn't come easy in the beginning.

- *Deep Breathing*: perform this exercise 10 – 15 minutes several times per day.

  Lie on your left side with a pillow slightly under your right hip so as not to lie flat on your back. Close your eyes and empty your mind of all thoughts. Take a long, deep breath and visualize fresh, cool air entering your nose and filling your lungs. Think the word "peace" or "calm" with each breath.

  Hold each breath for three to five seconds and exhale slowly from your mouth thinking the word "stress" or "fear." Continue this pattern of breathing for approximately 10 minutes, keeping the process slow and steady.

  * Again, remember to breathe slowly and not to tighten your abdominal muscles.

- *Muscle Relaxation*: perform this exercise 15 - 20 minutes several times per day.

  Close your eyes and empty your mind of all thoughts. Progressively, tense and relax various muscle groups and allow the stress to drain from your body.

  o Make a tight fist with each hand; hold the fists tightly closed for five seconds and focus on muscle tension. Relax your fists and focus on their feeling warm and heavy now that they are relaxed. Silently repeat, "My hands are calm and relaxed."
  o Make the lower and upper arms, as well as your fists, tense for five seconds. Focus on these muscle sensations. Relax these muscles and focus on their feeling warm, heavy, and relaxed.
  o Tense your shoulders, neck, face, and jaw as well as your arms and fists. Follow the above instructions.
  o Add additional muscle groups progressively and continue with the same instructions. <u>Remember to avoid the abdominal area with the tightening and relaxation since this could put undue pressure on your uterus and cervix.</u>

o   Go through your body tensing and relaxing each muscle group twice. Leave time to notice the difference between the relaxed muscles and the tense ones.

    * Remember to breathe slowly and do not tighten your abdominal muscles.

- *Meditation*: perform this exercise for 10 - 20 minutes in the beginning and increase time as the technique becomes perfected.

Meditation has two significant components: 1) Helps to focus your mind by concentrating on your breathing, a repetitive word or phrase, and for some people focusing on an object; 2) Encourages non-judgment of thoughts that circulate through your mind during the relaxation process.   When first starting to meditate, staying focused and in control of your thoughts for more than a few seconds may be difficult, but that is understandable. Just keep trying to bring your mind back into focus. A few minutes of relaxation music played prior to starting your meditation exercise may help things flow a little more smoothly and aid in relaxation. If you find meditation difficult and an increase in stress, take a break and give it a try later.

Performing Meditation:

o   Create a quite space where no one will interrupt or disturb you.
o   If your doctor permits sitting up, sit upright in a comfortable chair, close your eyes, relax your muscles and breathe in and out slowly and naturally.
o   If not permitted to sit up, lie on your left side with a pillow slightly under the right hip, close your eyes and relax your muscles as much as possible. Breathe in and out slowly and naturally.
o   Focus on your breathing, an object, a word, or a phrase. With each breath in you will **think** of your particular focus object, word, or phrase and with each breath out you will **say** your particular focus object, word, or phrase. For example, with each breath in you would **think** calm and with each breath out you would **say** calm.
o   As thoughts enter your mind, acknowledge they are there and return to your focus object and try not to get frustrated with

74

unrelated thoughts popping into your mind. This type of diversion is normal and will decrease over time with practice.

o Continue meditating for 10 – 20 minutes.

* Remember to breathe slowly and not to tighten the abdominal muscles.

- *Guided Imagery and Visualization*: perform exercise for at least 10 – 15 minutes building on time as you become more proficient at the exercise.

The concept behind guided imagery and visualization is to use the mind's eye to visualize and create a special place that offers safety and relaxation by blocking out stressors of normal life. It allows escaping to a place of your own creation.

When developing your movie for guided imagery, you are in total control. If you don't like a particular image, thought or feeling, you can change it. For example, if you are imagining you are lying on a beach in Jamaica with sounds of the birds and waves of the ocean surrounding you and, suddenly, something that brings stress into your life pops into your mind, you can visually imagine putting the person, place, or thing onto a raft and setting it afloat out to sea – never to bring stress into your life again. The goal is to have a special place inside your mind and heart that you can retreat to for safety and relaxation.

To enhance your guided imagery experience, you can move beyond just visual imagery to include your other senses such as smell, touch, taste, and sound.

Performing Guided Imagery and Visualization:

o Close your eyes and take several slow deep breaths in through your nose and exhale from your mouth.
o Think of a place that feels safe and comfortable for you. It can be real or imagined.
o Give yourself time to create the different aspects of your safe place. Piece by piece create a scene in your mind that feels calming and peaceful.

o   Once your image starts developing, take a good look around at the different aspects of your safe and relaxing place. Look from left to right, top to bottom, and front to back. Take in all the images slowly.

o   Allow yourself to enjoy your creation: sounds, colors, textures, and shapes.

o   Stop and listen for sounds in your special place. Listen for the wind, the birds, waves gently lapping onto the shores, and leaves rustling in the wind.

o   Allow yourself to feel the physical aspects of your creation – maybe the wind against your face, your clothing blowing in the wind, the wetness of the sand between your toes, etc.

o   In your mind's eye, allow yourself to touch some of the things in your special place. Maybe a leaf that has fallen onto the ground – feel it crumble between your fingers; enjoy a gentle rain falling onto your face.

o   Take in a deep breath inhaling through your nose, becoming aware of the smells accompanying the breath. Exhale from your mouth while thinking, "This is my special safe place where there is no worry or stress, just relaxation and peace."

o   When you are ready to leave your special place, take a deep breath, inhaling through your nose and exhaling fully from your mouth.

o   Open your eyes and just BE for a few minutes. Think about the special things from the place you created and savor that time of carefree living.

Continue to build on your special place or create new places each time you perform guided imagery and relaxation. You are in charge!

Learning to relax is certainly a skill and one worth honing. The above listed relaxation exercises will provide direction and motivation in helping to find the special relaxation technique that brings peace and comfort to your life.

Positive Thinking

As I sit here writing this section on positive thinking, I'm reminded of a conversation I had with a colleague while I was on bedrest. She called to offer her support and remind me that positive thinking would make my bedrest challenges less frightening. She proceeded to tell me all that I "should" be grateful for and how to think positively. After our conversation, I felt anything but positive. However, after thinking about our conversation, one thing she said really stood out to me, "Positive thinking would make my bedrest challenges less frightening." She reminded me of an important concept that I had lost sight of during my pregnancy crisis: the power of positive thinking.

Thinking positively about a life event can make all the difference in the world in how you think, feel, and respond. Just as negative thinking is a learned behavior, so is positive thinking. After we are born, we learn how to think about life events from behavior modeled to us from significant others in our lives, as well as from our own life experiences. We create a basic pattern of how we respond and think throughout our own development.

The goal of this section is to encourage you to evaluate how you think; to determine if your thinking process is mostly positive or negative; and to make a conscious choice about how you will continue processing information, especially your pregnancy bedrest experience.

Optimistic thinking has many benefits to health - both physical and emotional. Thinking positively can improve your mood and self-esteem; decrease depression, anxiety, and anger; reduce pain and muscle tension; and increase your immune system functioning. These are all very import aspects of healthy and happy living. To determine your particular type of thinking, you must begin with an honest appraisal about your thinking of self and of others. Ask yourself the hard questions and answer them candidly. The following are some questions to pose to yourself:

- Am I looking at pregnancy bedrest as punishment?
- Do I lie here most of the day thinking about all the things that have gone wrong and could go wrong?
- Am I overly critical of other people's comments and suggestions by thinking they have no idea what I am going through; how dare they offer me advice?
- Do I focus on the past and negative events that have taken place?
- Is my conversation more negative than positive in content?
- Do I look for the positive in situations, or jump straight to the negative?
- Am I over reactive to situations and give exaggerated responses?
- Do I think mostly in black and white (good or bad), or can I find shades of gray?

77

- Can I find positive things about my personality, or does the negative outweigh the positive in my mind?
- Do I over-worry about things? Do I spend a lot of time worrying about things that never happen?
- Do I have catastrophic thinking – assuming the worst will happen?
- Do I jump to conclusions before weighing the evidence?

These are questions you can start with to get an insight into your thinking. Keep in mind, change comes from the acceptance of the need for change.

Once you document your answers, put them aside and think about something else for awhile. Later, go back and ask yourself the questions again and see how your answers compare to the first time around. Initially, people tend to be more reserved in their responses. After a practice time or two, it seems easier to express your thoughts more openly. Once you have answers to the hard questions, you will be able to determine if your thinking tends to be pessimistic or optimistic. The next step in this "self-thinking evaluation exercise" is to determine if you want change. Once you determine a change is in order, start replacing those negative thoughts with positive ones, keeping in mind you have to become cognizant of your self-talk. This is where change begins - usually subtly and grows more consciously. The following are some examples of reframing from negative to positive.

Negative: My life is turned upside down. I can't lie in bed day after day – I will lose me mind.
Positive: Things have changed as a result of my pregnancy complications and I am going to make the best of them – at least my baby is safe. I will find different things I enjoy to occupy my time each day.

Negative: She is only calling to check on me because she feels obligated.
Positive: It was really nice to talk on the telephone for a few minutes today and to get to share how I am feeling. It feels good to know someone is thinking about me.

Negative: I know I won't make it to 36 weeks before the baby is born.

Positive: My goal for bedrest it to make it to 36 weeks gestation – that will be the number in my mind and I will do all I can to meet my goal.

Negative: Jeff has it so easy; he gets to go to work all day and talk with friends while I have to lie in bed all day.

Positive: I am so glad my husband has a good job to support us during this time so I don't have to worry about finances while on bedrest.

The goal is to weed out negative thinking and reframe it into positive thinking. Does this mean you will never have negative thoughts again; NO! We all have negative thoughts; however, it's what we do with the thoughts that count. Becoming aware of your negativism and how it is affecting your life and that of others is an opportunity to grow and learn more about who you are and who you want to become. Learning to focus on the positive aspects of life, especially when on pregnancy bedrest, will make for a happier, healthier, and more peaceful you. When we choose to look at a challenge as an opportunity for growth, growth will happen. If we choose to look at a challenge as getting the better of us, then we have become defeatists. The adage "you feel what you think" is very true. Learning to think positive will help you to feel positive, thus decreasing fear, anxiety, anger, depression, and other emotions that create stress surrounding your bedrest time. Having a positive outlook will help make your bedrest journey more manageable.

Chapter Seven

Exercises for Pregnancy Bedrest Maintaining Energy and Decreasing Muscle Strain

❧❧❧❧❧❧❧❧❧❧

Prior to pregnancy, I was a physically active person, running approximately six miles per week and performing high-impact aerobics two times per week. After becoming pregnant, I reduced my level of physical activity to a safer range of exercises per my OB/GYN's recommendation. When prescribed bedrest, I thought, "I'm physically fit; bedrest shouldn't affect my strength and muscle mass very much." I was wrong! Within four to five weeks, I was noticing a decrease in energy and strength and an increase in physical pain and stiffness. Fortunately, my doctor also noticed the change, and requested I be visited by a physical therapist who developed a daily pregnancy bedrest exercise routine for me.

While I was not able to maintain my normal fitness level, I was able to minimize muscle weakness, stiffness, and strain experienced by bedrest patients. Exercise also helped in preventing conditions brought on by poor blood circulation, including deep vein clots in the legs, reduction in blood flow to the uterus and baby, feeling light-headed, shortness of breath, and restlessness. In addition to the physical benefits of exercise, I benefited emotionally as well. Exercise helps to reduce stress, anxiety, and to balance mood, bringing about a more positive outlook. Therefore, a simple and safe exercise routine for pregnancy bedrest may be a good option. Prior to performing any exercises listed in this book or elsewhere, get your doctor's permission. Your own doctor's permission is imperative. Each woman's pregnancy condition is peculiar to her. What might be an acceptable exercise routine for one woman may not be for another. Remember, the goal is to keep you and your baby safe; please consult your doctor first!

Getting Started

- Start off slowly to determine your body's response to an increase in activity.
- DO NOT hold your breath. Inhale through your nose and exhale from your mouth, keeping your breathing at a normal, comfortable pace.
- DO NOT push or bear down. Avoid using your abdominal muscles for any of these exercises unless your doctor says it's okay.
- Keep your water container close by while exercising and drink occasionally to ensure you are not dehydrating your body.
- Exercise at a slow pace keeping movements smooth and simple. Discontinue any exercise that is uncomfortable, painful, or causes shortness of breath.
- Monitor your baby's response to exercise and stop if you have questions or concerns.
- When performing exercises, place a small pillow or rolled towel under the right hip. DO NOT lie flat on your back because doing so can impede blood flow to the uterus and increase contractions.
- Discontinue exercising and contact your doctor immediately if you notice a change in contractions, discharge from the vagina (blood or amniotic fluid), rapid heart rate, elevated blood pressure, back pain, dizziness, or increase in fluid retention.
- Tailor your exercise routine to your endurance level and pregnancy condition. Start out slowly and increase in duration as your body and doctor permit.

Pregnancy Bedrest Exercises

The following exercises are designed to keep muscles toned and to minimize weakness, strain, pain, and stiffness, as well as to improve blood circulation and emotional health. <u>Remember, you must have your doctor's approval before beginning any exercise routine</u>. Again, if at any time you start feeling discomfort or concern of any kind, discontinue exercises and contact your doctor.

Neck and Shoulders

- **Neck Stretch (5 - 10 repetitions)**

  Tuck your chin towards your chest and slowly roll your head from left to right holding each position 3 to 5 seconds, then return to the start position and maintain a chin tuck while pressing your head backwards into the pillow and holding it there for 3 to 5 seconds.

- **Shoulder Shrugs and Rolls (5 - 10 repetitions)**

  Shrug your shoulders bringing them up toward your ears. The shoulders can be moved at the same time or individually. After shoulder shrugs, roll both shoulders forward in a circle and then backward in a circle. Finish by pinching the shoulders together and releasing.

Hands, Wrists, and Arms

- **Finger Extension and Flexion (5 - 10 repetitions)**

  Hold your hand out in front of you, extend your fingers open as far as possible and hold for 5 seconds. Close fingers together and make a tight fist, hold for 5 seconds and release.

- **Thumb Finger Touch (5 - 10 repetitions)**

  Hold your wrist straight and form the letter "O" by gently touching your thumb to each fingertip. After each "O" straighten and spread your fingers.

- **Hand Shake (5 - 10 repetitions)**

  Drop your hands to your side and shake them gently as if you were shaking off droplets of water. This exercise can be done while sitting down or during a bathroom break.

- **Stress Ball Squeeze (3 – 5 repetitions)**

  With the palm of the hand facing up, place a soft foam ball in the palm and gently squeeze, holding for 5 seconds and release. This exercise will help to keep your hands strong and flexible, as well as provide stress relief. Be sure not to tense your shoulders during this exercise.

- ○ **Wrist Extension and Flexion (5 - 10 repetitions)**

  With your arm resting on a table (lap table when in bed), hang your hand off the end of the table with the wrist bent down until the sensation of stretching is felt. Hold this motion for 5 seconds and slowly return to the start position. Bend the same wrist in an upward motion until the sensation of stretching is felt. Hold this position for 5 seconds and return to the start position.

- ○ **Arm Stretches and Lifts (5 - 10 repetitions for each exercise)**

  1. Stretch one arm at a time down toward the knees, make a fist, release the fist and bend the elbow.
  2. Stretch one arm at a time up toward the ceiling and then back down to your side.
  3. Hold one arm out at a time in front of you and make large letters as if writing in the air.

  (If your doctor approves, these exercises can be done with wrist weights or hand weights.)

Legs, Ankles and Feet

- ○ **Legs (5 - 10 repetitions of each exercise)**

  During these exercises, keep a small pillow or rolled towel under your right hip so as not to lie flat on your back. Keep one hand on the abdomen to ensure you are not tightening your abdominal muscles and remember to take slow deep breaths!

  1. Bend your leg at the hip and knee. This movement will form the shape of a triangle with the bed being the base of the triangle. Keep your heel flat on the bed and extend your leg straight out, causing your leg to rest on the bed. Slowly move the extended leg back to the start position and repeat this exercise with the other leg.
  2. Lie on the bed with your legs straight and bend your right leg so your right heel sits flat on the bed. Take your right heel and

place it on top of your left ankle. Allow your right knee to rest out on its side and gently slide your right foot up your left leg until it makes contact with your knee. Then, gently slide the leg back down to the left ankle. Repeat this exercise with your opposite leg.

3. With your legs still straight and lying on the bed, gently roll your knees inward and outward.

4. With your legs straight and lying on the bed, press the back of your knees into the bed, tightening your thigh muscles. Hold this position for 5 seconds and release. Both legs can be tightened at the same time. Repeat this exercise 10 times remembering to breathe and not to tighten abdominal muscles.

5. Bend your knees slightly and dig your heels into the bed. Hold this position for 5 seconds and release. Both legs can be exercised at the same time or one at a time. Repeat the exercise 10 times, remembering to breathe and not to tighten the abdominal muscles.

○ **Ankle Pumps and Foot Rotations (10 – 15 repetitions several times daily)**

1. With your legs resting on the bed, gently move your foot (or both feet) with a pumping motion as though pressing the gas peddle to accelerate a car and then letting off the gas peddle. This exercise can also be performed with exercise bands when permitted by your doctor.

2. With your legs resting on the bed, gently rotate your feet in a clockwise motion and then counter-clockwise motion.

Maintaining Energy and Decreasing Muscle Strain

Pregnancy bedrest can zap energy quickly and subject the body to muscle strain. The following tips will help maintain safety and health.

- When lying in bed, always try to keep the spine as straight as possible. This will help with reduction in muscle strain.
- Lying on the left side is the best position for blood flow to the uterus and to the baby and should be done as much as can be tolerated; however, all of us who have done long stints of bedrest know that rotating sides is necessary because of joint pain and stiffness. When lying on your side, place a pillow under your

neck, behind your back, between your knees, and slightly under your stomach. The extra pillows will provide added support to the spine and help with reduction in muscle strain. Note: a body pillow is a great investment!

- When moving from side to side in the bed, keep your head on a pillow and roll like a log. This move helps to keep the spine straight and prevents pressure on the abdomen and cervix.
- When attempting to sit up in bed, roll to one side and bring the legs to the edge of the bed prior to pushing up with the arms. After your legs are at the edge of the bed, use both arms to push yourself up to a sitting position while you swing your legs over the edge of the bed. Reverse this motion when lying back down. NEVER attempt to sit straight up as this will force you to tighten your abdominal muscles and apply pressure to the uterus and cervix.
- When attempting to sit up in a hospital bed, keep your head on the pillow and raise the head of your electric bed.
- Always sit on the edge of the bed for a few seconds before walking around since rising too quickly can cause lightheadedness. Take 3 deep slow breaths and straighten and bend each leg before getting up from the bed.
- When moving about the house to shower, use the bathroom, or perform other chores, take it slow and easy. It's not uncommon for a person to feel lightheaded when moving to an upright position and walking around after being in bed for extended periods of time.
- When sitting up or moving about, remember the importance of good posture. You are growing each day and your muscles are weakening more each day and poor posture can cause additional muscle strain.

By doing all you can to stay healthy, you are giving yourself and your baby a gift. After bedrest is over, you will be back on your feet, and these exercises will help to make the transition into normal life a little smoother and less painful.

Chapter Eight

Spiritual Reflection
Tending Your Spiritual Garden
Words of Inspiration

✤✤✤✤✤✤✤✤✤✤✤

When in the midst of a crisis or difficult life situation, we sometimes find ourselves pondering the deeper meaning of life and of life's experiences. Further, we explore the various aspects of our humanness by seeking understanding and answers to questions in the hopes of lessening our pain, grief, and worry. I found myself in this very situation when I faced pregnancy bedrest. "Why is my life's journey leading me in this direction?" "Am I a strong enough person to handle a negative outcome?" These questions, plus many more, were thoughts I pondered daily. I couldn't make sense of why everything that I had hoped for during the last two years of my life was on the verge of being taken from me.

While searching my heart and mind for answers, I was reminded of a conversation with one of my professors, while I was attending seminary earning my masters degree in marriage and family therapy. A group of us were discussing spirituality and spiritual reflection, when the professor shared with us a life struggle he had endured. His ten year old son had been killed while riding a bicycle. After his son's death, the professor communicated that he felt like a lost man emotionally and spiritually. Everything he had known and loved had been ripped out of his life and had brought with it questioning, especially about his faith. While he still had his wife and daughter, he was unable to see past his grief and his pain to feel the love they shared with and for him. A deep, dark abyss is how he depicted his existence. At no time in his life had he ever experienced this type of emotional and spiritual distress.

One of the students asked, "What about your faith in God; was that not a solace?" He smiled and said, "You don't understand – I blamed God for my pain. I was a man looking for meaning and understanding and there were no acceptable answers to why my son was taken from me."

Another student responded, "God didn't take your son, a man in a car who chose to exercise his right to free will and behave in a negative manner took your son." The professor responded, "That's exactly the answer I would have given to someone telling me this story, until I had my own life experience. We are humans and we need answers to the hard questions. We may never get them, yet we seek them. We want someone to blame when we are hurt and lost, its human nature."

Another student asked, "How did you start your spiritual healing journey?" The professor responded, "I was looking into the mirror at my face one morning and could feel nothing but sadness. It felt as if I were looking at an empty man – just a shell and all alone. With no direction or concrete thoughts I prayed for strength."

As time passed, he began feeling better emotionally; however, he still struggled with a sense of emptiness. He confided in a colleague about his struggles and she asked him, "How's your garden doing?" His response was, "I don't have a garden." She responded, "Yes, you do, and you have been neglecting it; that's where your emptiness lies." He walked out of her office angry. He mulled over her comment for several weeks and decided she was right – he had not been tending his "spiritual garden."

The question in his mind was "Can I face the deepest part of my being and survive all that will come with it?" He soon realized he didn't have a choice if he were ever to find the direction he so needed to face every day without his son. Through tears, he said "I looked through the window of my soul and saw a man worth saving." He had found the courage to journey to the center of his humanness – his spirit. He realized his spirit had been wounded too; spiritual healing had begun.

I will forever be grateful for his educating my spirit and giving me courage to take my own spiritual reflection journey. I have reflected on that conversation during difficult times in my own life and have found hope and strength. When faced with a medically challenged pregnancy, it's normal for any woman and her partner alike, to find him or herself struggling with the deeper meaning of life. Not knowing for sure if things are going to turn out positively or negatively is a difficult reality to face. Sometimes worry can get the best of us, bringing with it feelings of fear, anger, sadness, and depression. However, being able to journey to the deepest part of our existence, our spirit, and finding peace and hope can be invaluable when facing a crisis such as pregnancy bedrest. As there is healing for the physical and emotional aspects of our humanness, there is healing for spiritual woundedness as well.

In sharing this story with you, I hope you discover the courage and the desire to find spiritual healing if you are struggling with that aspect of your life. This is not to say that bedrest is a good time to take on emotional and spiritual journeys that may cause distress because you have enough stress, but an insight to inner feelings gives encouragement to allow yourself joy, peace, and hope.

Tending Your Spiritual Garden

Learning to nurture one's spirit should rank up there with nurturing one's body and mind. If we are to address the completeness of self, we cannot ignore our spiritual development. The spirit must be nurtured. This is not to say a particular religion must be followed, but do realize there are three aspects to your humanness: physical, emotional, and spiritual, and each affects the other. When on bedrest, the physical tending is obvious, you follow your doctor's orders: limit your activities as directed, eat in a healthy manner for your pregnancy condition, and take your medication, among other dictates. Emotionally, you will struggle with aspects of change, and you will work on ways to deal with these changes that are healthy for you and your family. The spirit, however, can be left unattended when overshadowed by the physical and emotional tending. Therefore, I invite you to set aside time to experience and enjoy moments of spiritual reflection during this difficult journey. My message is not to say open up wounds which might cause distress and possibly affect your pregnancy condition negatively, but rather work to process your current situation and determine if your spiritual garden needs a little extra tending as a result of the issues brought about by pregnancy bedrest.

A healthy, positive spirit brings peace, comfort, guidance, faith, knowledge, and love. Many experiences throughout life will be ones that only you can understand in your heart and mind, and one of those experiences is the pregnancy bedrest journey. Having a place inside you that is hopeful, peaceful, nurturing, and guiding will be strength to draw from when experiencing life struggles.

So, the question is "How do I tend my spiritual garden (a place of hope, peace, nurture, and guidance) so it can flourish?" The answer will vary from person to person. Tending ones spiritual garden is an ongoing learning experience particular to each life experience. How I tend my spiritual garden may not work for you, therefore, knowing who you are and what you need will help you on this journey. Particular to me, I set aside time daily to tend my spiritual garden by fertilizing it with meditation and relaxation time. Clearing my mind and experiencing the feeling of just being helps me to appreciate who I am and provides reflection time as to who I want to become. I think about the things I am grateful for and reflect on how much I have grown out of my times of struggle. Once the fertilization process is complete, I water my garden with inspiring quotes to help me grow in a direction that is positive and life giving. After each gardening expedition, I feel a little more complete.

In chapter six, I have provided information pertaining to relaxation and meditation and the different techniques that aid in relaxing. This will be a good starting point to your embarking on a spiritual reflection journey. Additionally, I am sharing my "wellspring" of quotes that bring inspiration and direction to my own life. As you read through these quotes, take note of certain ones that stand out for you. The ones that stand out most for you are probably the ones you most need at this particular time in your journey. Allow your mind to nurture your spirit by exploring the feelings stirred from the quotes that seem significant to you. Ask yourself the question "What do I feel when I read this particular quote and what do I need?" Write your answers down and take time to process the significance of your thoughts and feelings. After processing your thoughts and feelings, implement healthy coping and nurturing strategies for change that provide relief and direction.

Words of Inspiration and Direction

Faith & Hope

Faith is taking the first step even when you don't see the whole staircase.

~ *Martin Luther King, Jr.*

The best and most beautiful things in the world cannot be seen or even touched. They must be felt with the heart.

~ *Helen Keller*

Every tomorrow has two handles. We can take hold of it with the handle of anxiety or the handle of faith.

~ *Henry Ward Beecher*

When one door of happiness closes, another opens.

~ *Helen Keller*

Were it not for hope the heart would break.

~ *Scottish Proverb*

We must accept finite disappointment, but we must never lose infinite hope.

~ *Martin Luther King, Jr.*

Faith is the strength by which a shattered world shall emerge into the light.

~ *Helen Keller*

Hope sees the invisible, feels the intangible, and achieves the impossible.

~ *Author Unknown*

Hope is the thing with feathers – that perches in the soul – and sings a tune without words – and never stops, at all.

~ *Emily Dickinson*

What oxygen is to the lungs, such is hope to the meaning of life.

~ *Emil Brunner*

What seems impossible one minute becomes, through faith, possible the next.

~*Norman Vincent Peale*

Positive Thinking

Adopting the right attitude can convert a negative stress into a positive one.

~ *Hans Selye*

Worry doesn't empty tomorrow of its sorrows. It empties today of its strength.

~ *Author Unknown*

At the center of our agency is our freedom to form a healthy attitude toward whatever circumstances we are placed in!

~ *Neal A. Maxwell*

Ability is what you're capable of doing. Motivation determines what you do. Attitude determines how well you do it.

~ *Lou Holtz*

A man is what he thinks about all day long.

~ *Ralph Waldo Emerson*

There is little difference in people, but that little difference makes a big difference. That little difference is attitude. The big difference is whether it is positive or negative.

~ *W. Clement Stone*

Courage is not the absence of fear, but rather the judgment that something else is more important than fear.

~ *Ambrose Redmoon*

Positive anything is better than negative nothing.

~ *Elbert Hubbard*

A great pleasure in life is doing what people say you cannot do.

~ *Walter Bagehot*

No pessimist ever discovered the secret of the stars, or sailed to an uncharted land, or opened a new doorway for the human spirit.

~ *Helen Keller*

Difficulties are meant to rouse, not discourage. The human spirit is to grow strong by conflict.

~*William Ellery Channing*

Don't go through life, grow through life.

~ *Eric Butterworth*

Patience & Perseverance

Self-pity is our worst enemy and if we yield to it, we can never do anything wise in the world.

~ *Helen Keller*

Life's up and downs provide windows of opportunity to determine your values and goals. Think of using all obstacles as stepping stones to build the life you want.

~ *Marsha Sinetar*

It still holds true that man is most uniquely human when he turns obstacles into opportunities.

~ *Eric Hoffer*

It is not what we take up, but what we give up, that makes us rich.

~ *Henry Ward Beecher*

Many people have the wrong idea of what constitutes true happiness. It is not attained through self-gratification but through fidelity to a worthy purpose.

~ *Helen Keller*

Courage is being afraid but going on anyhow.

~ *Dan Rather*

Stand up to your obstacles and do something about them. You will find that they haven't half the strength you think they have.

~ *Norman Vincent Peale*

Defeat never comes to any man until he admits it.

~ *Josephus Daniels*

It is inevitable that some defeat will enter even the most victorious life. The human spirit is never finished when it is defeated…it is finished when it surrenders.

~ *Ben Stein*

Determination, patience and courage are the only things needed to improve any situation.

~ *Author Unknown*

Even a happy life cannot be without a measure of darkness, and the word happy would lose its meaning if it were not balanced by sadness. It is far better to take things as they come along with patience and equanimity.

~ *Carl Jung*

Learn to relax. Your body is precious, as it houses your mind and spirit. Inner peace begins with a relaxed body.

~ *Norman Vincent Peale*

Only those who have the patience to do simple things perfectly will acquire the skill to do difficult things easily.

~ *Johann Friedrich von Schiller*

Patience and perseverance have a magical effect before which difficulties disappear and obstacles vanish.

~ John Quincy Adams

Press on. Obstacles are seldom the same size tomorrow as they are today.

~ Robert H. Schuller

Spiritual Encouragement

The wealth of a soul is measured by how much it can feel; its poverty by how little.

~William R. Alger

People are like stained glass windows. They sparkle and shine when the sun is out, but when the darkness sets in; their true beauty is revealed only if there is a light from within.

~Elizabeth Kubler-Ross

Every trial endured and weathered in the right spirit makes a soul nobler and stronger than it was before.

~ James Buckham

Miracles, in the sense of phenomena we cannot explain, surround us on every hand; life itself is the miracle of miracles.

~ George Bernard Shaw

Expect the dawn of a new beginning in the dark nights of life.

~Lloyd John Ogilvie

Miracles happen to those who believe in them.

~Bernhard Berenson

When we lose one blessing, another is often, most unexpectedly, given in its place.

~ C.S. Lewis

Depression loses its power when fresh vision pierces the darkness.

~ Peter Sinclair

Man is so made that when anything fires his soul, impossibilities vanish.

~ Jean De La Fontaine

There are only two ways to live your life. One is though nothing is a miracle. The other is as though everything is a miracle.

~ *Albert Einstein*

It is only possible to live happily ever after on a day to day basis.

~ *Margaret Bonnano*

Joy is the feeling of grinning on the inside.

~ *Dr. Melba Colgrove*

Out of difficulties grow miracles.

~ *Jean De La Bruyere*

One joy scatters a hundred grieves.

~ *Chinese Proverb*

Not in rewards, but in the strength to strive, the blessing lies.

~ *J.T. Towbridge*

What seem to us bitter trials are often blessings in disguise.

~ *Oscar Wilde*

It is always wise to stop wishing for things long enough to enjoy the fragrance of those now flowering.

~ *Patrice Gifford*

Impossible situations can become possible miracles.

~ *Robert H. Schuller*

Love, Laughter and Friendship

We are all born for love. It is the principle of existence, and its only end.

~ *Benjamin Disraeli*

The only way to love anything is to realize that it might be lost.

~ *G.K. Chesterton*

Against the assault of laughter nothing can stand.

~ *Mark Twain*

Where there are friends, there is wealth.

~ *Titus Muccius Plautus*

You will find, as you look back upon your life, that the moments when you really lived are the moments when you have done things in the spirit of love.

~ *Henry Drummond*

Love changes darkness into light and makes the heart take a wingless flight.

~ *Helen Steiner Rice*

When we hurt each other we should write it down in the sand, so the winds of forgiveness can make it go away for good. When we help each other we should chisel it in stone, lest we never forget the love of a friend.

~ *Christian H. Godefroy*

Love is a fruit in season at all times, and within the reach of every hand.

~ *Mother Teresa*

How rare and wonderful is that flash of a moment when we realize we have discovered a friend.

~ *William E. Rothschild*

Laughter is an instant vacation.

~ *Milton Berle*

Laughter is the greatest weapon we have and we, as humans, use it the least.

~ *Mark Twain*

You can make more friends in two months by becoming interested in other people than you can in two years by trying to get other people interested in you.

~ *Dale Carnegie*

Love cures people – both the ones who give it and the ones who receive it.

~ *Dr. Karl Menninger*

What we have once enjoyed we can never lose. All that we love deeply becomes a part of us.

~ *Helen Keller*

I awoke with devout thanksgiving for my friends.

~ *Ralph Waldo Emerson*

Where there is great love there is always miracles.

~ *Willa Cather*

Laughter is the sun that drives winter from the human face.

~ *Victor Hugo*

We cannot tell the precise moment when friendship is formed. As in filling a vessel drop by drop, there is at last a drop which makes it run over. So in a series of kindness there is, at last, one which makes the heart run over.

~ *James Bowell*

Laughter is not a bad beginning for a friendship, and it is the best ending for one.

~ *Henry Ward Beecher*

Treat your friends as you do your pictures, and place them in their best light.

~ *Jennie Jerome Churchill*

Anger and Forgiveness

He who angers you conquers you.

~ *Elizabeth Kenny*

Anger ventilated often hurries toward forgiveness; and concealed often hardens into revenge.

~ *Edward G. Gulwe-Lytton*

For every minute you are angry, you lose sixty seconds of happiness.

~ *Author Unknown*

Forgiveness is a funny thing. It warms the heart and cools the sting.

~ *William Arthur Ward*

If you are angry at a loved one, hug that person. And mean it. You may not want to hug – which is all the more reason to do so. It's hard to stay angry when someone shows they love you, and that's precisely what happens when we hug each other.

~ *Walter Anderson*

Don't let anger weaken your internal flame.

~ *Author Unknown*

Forgive all who have offended you, not for them, but for yourself.

~ *Harriet Nelson*

Get mad then get over it.

~ *Colin Powell*

I don't have to attend every argument I'm invited to.

~ *Author Unknown*

Holding onto anger is like grasping a hot coal with the intent of throwing it at someone else; you are the one who gets burned.

~ *Buddha*

Consider how much more you often suffer from your anger and grief, than from those very things for which you are angry and grieved.

~ *Marcus Antonius*

When you hold resentment toward another, you are bound to that person or condition by an emotional link that is stronger than steel. Forgiveness is the only way to dissolve that link and get free.

~ *Catherine Ponder*

There is no revenge so complete as forgiveness.

~ *Josh Billings*

Mothers and Children

A baby is a kiss from heaven blown from the hand of God.

~ *Author Unknown*

Fear not for tomorrow. God is already there.

~ *Author Unknown*

A mother understands what a child does NOT say.

~ *Jewish Proverb*

Think of stretch marks as pregnancy service stripes.

~ *Joyce Armor*

Biology is the least of what makes someone a mother.

~ *Oprah Winfrey*

A baby is an angel whose wings decrease as his legs increase.

~ *Author Unknown*

As a mother, I must faithfully, patiently, lovingly and happily do my part – then quietly wait for God to do His.

~ *Ruth Bell Graham*

A mother is a person who seeing there are only four pieces of pie for five people, promptly announces she never did care for pie.

~ *Tenneva Jordan*

Perhaps the greatest social service that can be rendered by anybody to the country and to mankind is to bring up a family.

~ *George Bernard Shaw*

A mother never quite leaves her children at home, even when she doesn't take them along.

~ *Margaret Culkin Banning*

We find delight in the beauty and happiness of children that makes the heart too big for the body.

~ *Ralph Waldo Emerson*

God's interest in the human race is nowhere better evidenced than in obstetrics.

~ *Martin H. Fisher*

It is easier to build strong children than to repair broken men.

~ *Frederick Douglas*

A mother is one to whom you hurry when you are troubled.

~ *Emily Dickinson*

Mother's love is peace. It need not be acquired, it need not be deserved.

~ Erich Fromm

A baby is God's opinion that the world should go on.

~ Carl Sandburg

Mother is the name for God in the lips and hearts of little children.

~ William Makepeace Thackeray

Youth fades; love droops; the leaves of friendship fall; a mother's secret hope outlives them all.

~ Oliver Wendell Holmes

Having a child is surely the most beautifully irrational act that two people in love can commit.

~ Bill Cosby

Chapter Nine

Days Following Pregnancy Bedrest
Types of Postpartum Challenges
Taking Charge of Your Postpartum Depression
Postpartum Depression Support Contacts

֍֍֍֍֍֍֍֍֍֍֍

When approaching the end of pregnancy bedrest, the excitement for the expectant mother becomes immeasurable. "Finally, I get to have a normal life again," was my thought. I had a plan for all the things I wanted to do, in what restaurant I wanted to dine, and which stores I wanted to shop. Boy, was I fooling myself! The bedrest journey was over, and a new journey had started – recouping from fourteen weeks in bed. My body was physically exhausted. I remember my doctor telling me to resume normal activities, and I did try. However, resuming normal activities was not an easy task; in fact, it took some time. So, when the bedrest journey is over; take it slow. Your mind may want to go, but the body needs time to catch up.

Try not to get frustrated about your physical endurance level because it will increase. Continue your bedrest exercises during this post bedrest period and add others that your doctor approves. After the baby arrives and you get through your six week postpartum time frame, you will be able to design an exercise plan that will restore energy and strength. In the meantime, a lot of stretching will be beneficial, especially for the back, neck, arms, legs, ankles, and feet. After bedrest, one of my biggest difficulties, besides fatigue, was ankle pain. After the body has been supine for long periods of time, the Achilles tendon can shorten and weaken, bringing about intense pain when walking. My ankle pain didn't begin immediately after getting off bedrest, but did set in several weeks later. I didn't realize I needed to be stretching these tendons, as well as my knee and elbow tendons daily as my activity level was increasing, so keep this complication in mind. After about two months, I could tell a huge difference in my energy and strength. It all does come back; it just takes time. So, remember to take it slow and to keep yourself safe.

On a different note, I feel it is important to examine another challenge that many women experience after pregnancy: postpartum depression. Reflecting on the first few weeks after Lydia's birth, I'm reminded of my own personal struggles with postpartum depression. My feelings of parenting were mixed. I was happy to be a mom and grateful for my pregnancy outcome, but I struggled with feelings of being overwhelmed in my new role. I was physically exhausted from fourteen weeks in bed, breastfeeding was not going well, and I was recovering from an unplanned c-section. Lydia was a normal infant with many demands, and I wanted to meet all of them; however, I had moments of feeling as if I had no more to give. Additionally, I was struggling with feelings of shame and inadequacy. I had allowed myself to fall into the mythical thinking of being a "perfect mother." I knew there was no such creature; however, I wanted my afterbirth story to look and feel as easy as other mother's had seemed. I remember one afternoon when a girlfriend came by for a visit. She, too, had a new baby who was two weeks older than Lydia. My friend reported how well breastfeeding was going and how well her daughter was sleeping and napping. To top things off, she expressed how helpful her mother had been by taking care of the daughter every Saturday night for a few hours, so she and her husband could have a date night. She seemed intoxicated with her role as a mother. She was on a carousel ride experiencing only the wonders of motherhood. Then, there was me who felt like the horse with spaghetti legs on a carousel and about to collapse.

After my friend left that afternoon, I remember feeling jealous that she had family near by to help her out, and that motherhood seemed so easy for her. I remember thinking "What is wrong with me?" "Why am I struggling, and she isn't?" I was definitely in a self-defeating mode. Later that night while rocking Lydia to sleep, I took the time to look at my child, smell her baby scent, touch her soft skin and remind myself that all people are different and all respond to change in their own particular way. I told myself, "I am a good mother and I love my baby just as much as other mothers. Just because I am struggling some doesn't make me abnormal." This was a pivotal day for me. I broke out of my state of denial and acknowledged what I already knew in my heart and mind: I was struggling with symptoms of postpartum depression.

After putting Lydia to bed that night, I allowed myself the time to have a serious cry – you know "the ugly cry" when your lips are quivering, snot running down your face, and you are gasping for air. After letting out the emotions I had been bottling for several weeks, I made a promise to myself, "Beginning tomorrow I will start my postpartum depression journey with eyes of hope instead of despair; I want to enjoy this time of parenting."

I confided in Jon and explained to him that I was struggling with postpartum depression and what postpartum depression meant, and asked for his help in finding my way. He was my rock once again. Every evening he came home and took over caring for Lydia for a few hours so I could have time to myself for relaxation and rest. Just having those moments of "me time" helped enormously. In addition to relaxation and rest, I became very aware of what and when I ate, making sure I was getting the nutrients I needed, as well as cutting out consumption of refined sugar and caffeine. It wasn't long before I noticed a shift in energy and mood.

During my six week postpartum check-up, I spoke candidly with my doctor about my postpartum struggles. I remember expressing to her my feelings of shame in acknowledging I had postpartum depression, and she reminded me statistically that 70 to 80 percent of women experience some shift in mood after childbirth, and 10 to 20 percent of women experience some form of postpartum depression ranging from mild, to moderate, to severe. Also, she encouraged me to cut myself some slack. Her actual words were, "Goodness sakes, Wanda, you were in bed for fourteen weeks, endured an emergency c-section, and breastfeeding difficulties. Of course, you are going to have an adjustment period. Just being out of bed is a huge adjustment." And she was right. I had been through a lot. When I left her office that day, I felt very hopeful.

By ten week's postpartum, I was feeling much better. I'm glad my battle with postpartum depression was mild and short lived. However, some of my friends have not been as fortunate. Several experienced moderate postpartum depression which required antidepressants and therapy for several months. I am, however, very pleased to report they overcame their postpartum depression and are doing great today. My hope is that you will not have to endure postpartum depression. But, if you do, know you can get through it, and by all means, ask for help. Under no circumstance should you judge yourself negatively. You did not choose to have postpartum depression just as you didn't choose to have a medically challenged pregnancy that landed you on bedrest – it's just out of your control. However, treating postpartum depression is in your control. There is no need to suffer in silence when you don't have to do so. Certainly there is nothing to be ashamed of – you are a human being responding in your own particular way to change. We are all different, and thank goodness for that! I hope the information presented here will help provide education, support, and direction for you, should you struggle with postpartum depression issues after bedrest.

Types of Postpartum Challenges

The following are the three postpartum categories a woman might fall into after the birth of a child:

- *Baby Blues*: Immediately after a women goes through childbirth, her estrogen and progesterone hormones drop, which can bring on feelings of sadness, anxiety, increased sensitivity, laughing one minute and crying the next, anger, and other types of moodiness. Additionally, the hormones produced by the thyroid gland may drop sharply. The thyroid gland helps to regulate metabolism, which is how the body uses and stores energy from foods consumed. If the thyroid isn't functioning properly, the new mother may feel tired, sluggish, and depressed. Also, the amount of blood in the body, blood pressure, immune system, and metabolism all change after giving birth. These changes can affect how the mother feels physically and emotionally, causing fatigue and/or mood swings. When these physical changes occur, it's not uncommon for a woman to be diagnosed with the "baby blues." The baby blues period usually begins within a couple of days after child birth and diminishes within two weeks or so. The baby blues are very common with approximately 70-80 percent of women experiencing some symptoms after childbirth; however, the concern comes when the symptoms do not dissipate in two weeks or so – this could signal postpartum depression.

- *Postpartum Depression (PPD)*: Postpartum depression can range from mild, to moderate, to severe. To date, there is no exact answer to what causes a woman to experience postpartum depression, only theories. Regardless of the exact cause, we all know that postpartum depression exists and is more than a mental health issue as was once thought. Fortunately, doctors are now taking women's reports of physical, emotional, and behavioral changes after childbirth seriously.

- Postpartum depression can begin as early as a few days after childbirth or up to one year during the postpartum period. The following is a good list of symptoms.

  o Uncontrollable crying.

  o Anxiety and/or panic: this can be in the form of rapid heart rate, physical shaking, sweating, restlessness, uncontrollable fear, sense of doom, chest pain or pressure, dizziness, insomnia, need to disconnect from others either emotionally, and/or physically.

  o Feeling empty and sad: unable to experience joy or pleasure, including a loss of interest in activities which once brought pleasure.

  o Irritability and/or anger: this can be seen with strong responses to events or actions not deserving of a strong response.

  o Low self-esteem: feeling inadequate, unworthy, guilty, and helpless: negative self talk about your parenting abilities and desires to include fear and shame for your feelings.

  o Decrease in appetite or noticeable increase in appetite which affects you negatively.

  o Disturbance in sleep from reasons other than caring for an infant.

  o Loss of energy: constant fatigue or feeling as if "running on empty."

  o Isolation and/or loneliness: distancing yourself from friends, family, work, or children. Staying in the house all the time and/or fearing to leave the house thinking something may happen to you or the baby.

  o Poor grooming and hygiene behavior.

  o Difficulty concentrating, remembering, conversing, and making decisions.

  o Fear of being alone with the baby.

  o Thoughts of harming the baby, yourself, or someone else.

  o Feelings of rejection for your baby and/or other love ones.

  o Fear of being alone and/or being in the company of others.

  o Thoughts of running away to avoid responsibilities.

  o Overly concerned for baby (sense of paranoia).

  o Disorganized, resulting in the inability to perform simple, normal tasks to include multi-tasking.

- o Physical ailments with no known cause and no response to medical treatment, such as headaches, breathing difficulties, unexplained physical pain, and diarrhea.
- o Obsessive-compulsive behaviors: constantly checking on the baby or obsessing about the baby or other displays of obsessive-compulsive behavior such as counting numbers over and over in your mind, repetitive checking behavior, such as checking the stove to make sure it is off, time and time again, and checking the locks on the door to ensure the door is locked many times over.

- *Postpartum Psychosis*: Postpartum psychosis is a very rare condition and very serious. The onset of postpartum psychosis usually occurs within a few days after childbirth but can be delayed up to approximately three months after childbirth. Postpartum psychosis usually presents with the mother being out of touch with reality: hearing voices, seeing people who are not present, disorganized and/or bizarre thinking, and homicidal and/or suicidal impulses. From being out of touch with reality, a mother experiencing postpartum psychosis will need others to notice these changes and help her to get medical care. Medical care needs to be sought immediately when symptoms become noticeable; don't wait to see if the symptoms of postpartum psychosis will resolve on their own.

The following is a list of symptoms that MUST be addressed immediately for everyone's safety if postpartum psychosis is a possibility:

- o Paranoid behavior
- o Aggressive behavior
- o Severe depression
- o Hallucinations
- o Delusions
- o Bizarre behavior(s)
- o Irrational thoughts and behaviors
- o Threats or attempts of suicide or homicide

Taking Charge of Your Postpartum Depression

Pregnancy bedrest has been endured, and now you are faced with the struggles of postpartum depression. When will it ever end?! I know that was my thinking. However, just as with pregnancy bedrest, you will overcome. As I have said many times in this book, difficult experiences can make us stronger – we just have to find our route on the journey. The following list of self-care suggestions will help you find your route. Please keep in mind the importance of talking with your doctor about postpartum depression concerns. Help is there; you just have to reach out and accept it!

- Get as much rest as possible. When the baby takes a nap, take one too. Ask and accept help from others who are willing to help you get a few hours of down time.
- Try not to put a lot of pressure on yourself. Accept that you will do what you can and the rest will have to wait until another day.
- Do not over extend yourself by trying to do things for others. Doing so makes your struggles more difficult.
- Work out a plan with your mate regarding night time feeding schedules and chores. Ask everyone in the home to pitch in and help you out while you are getting back on your feet. Help is very important after coming off bedrest. Your body will be weak and take a harder hit with fatigue than the woman who was up and around during her pregnancy.
- Remind yourself that you are a good mother and that you love your baby.
- Watch your diet. Make sure you are eating healthy meals and snacks. It's easy to get caught up in parenting and realize it is noon and you still have not eaten breakfast. Also, limit your caffeine, sugar, and alcohol intake since stimulants and depressants can affect your mood and energy level.
- Exercise is a good way of helping the body balance itself. Once you have been given permission from your doctor to begin exercising again, get an exercise routine together that includes both cardio conditioning and weight training. Go slow at first, keeping in mind your recent pregnancy journey.
- Make sure you get out of the house at least a few minutes each day. It's easy to get in the mode of staying inside, and, before long, you end up feeling isolated. Try not to spend a lot of time alone.

- Shower and get dressed everyday, include hair care and make-up.
- Set aside time to listen to relaxation music as often as possible. This can be done in the home or in the car.
- Incorporate the relaxation exercises listed in this book into your postpartum recovery routine.
- Join support groups for women suffering from postpartum depression. Keep in mind the glass as a half full concept instead of a half empty one. It's certainly understandable to exchange stories, however, avoid getting caught in the victim competition.
- Schedule time alone with your mate to talk about what you are experiencing and how he is coping during this time. Most husbands want to help their wives feel better, so tell him what you need.
- Contact your church or other organization for support and possible connections with other women in your area dealing with postpartum depression.
- Don't allow yourself to get stuck in a "beat yourself up mode." Think of good things in your life and reframe the distressing things into more positive things.
- Seek professional treatment. Contact a local mental health organization and find someone who specializes in postpartum depression. Psychotherapy can help you realize necessary changes in behavior that could significantly impact your condition. This treatment will also provide you with a safe haven where you can be who you are and not have to worry about anyone else for an hour or so.
- Should you and your doctor agree that medication is necessary for the treatment of your postpartum depression, take it and see how you respond. Most physicians recommend SSRI's (selective serotonin reuptake inhibitors) to treat postpartum depression. SSRI's work by increasing the availability of the neurotransmitter serotonin in your brain. Many women have wonderful results with antidepressants in treating postpartum depression. On average, approximately four to six weeks are needed to feel the full therapeutic effect. However, some women notice improvements in mood within a few weeks. If you choose the antidepressant route, be sure your medication is closely monitored by your physician to ensure the most effective dosage and to minimize side effects. Read all the material provided that describe side effects and possible concerns of the medication. Should you have any concerns, discuss them with your doctor. If you are breastfeeding,

you will want your doctor to know because antidepressants are secreted in small amounts in breast milk.

My hope is that these suggestions will be beneficial to you during the postpartum period and will help you avoid or lessen the impact of post pregnancy issues. Remember, you have many life experiences to get through – this is just one. You will conquer these complications with determination and diligence. Just as pregnancy bedrest affects all involved, so does postpartum depression. Remember to love yourself, and to accept and respect yourself enough to get help because you deserve a new outlook on life. Reaching out for help shows strong character - not weak cowardice.

Postpartum Depression Support Contacts

The following is a list of organizations focused on helping women who are struggling during the postpartum period. If you have ANY questions pertaining to postpartum depression, do not hesitate to contact the folks at these organizations. They want to help. Also, keep in mind your own OB/GYN is a great resource for help with postpartum depression issues.

National Institute of Mental Health, NIH, HHS
Telephone: 301-496-9576
www.NIMH.NIH.GOV

National Mental Health Information Center, SAMHSA, HHS
Telephone: 800-789-2647
www.Mentalhealth.org

American Psychological Association
Telephone: 800-374-2721
www.apa.org

Postpartum Education for Parents
Telephone: 805-564-3888
www.SBPEP.org

Postpartum Support International
Telephone: 800-773-6667 or 805-967-7636
www.Postpartum.net

National Women's Health Information Center (NWHIC)
Telephone: 800-994-5446
www.4woman.gov/

American College of Obstetricians and Gynecologists (ACOG)
Telephone: 202-484-3321
www.ACOG.com

Resources for Education & Entertainment

≼ઈ≼ઈ≼ઈ≼ઈ≼ઈ≼ઈ≼ઈ≼ઈ≼ઈ≼ઈ

Completing the journey of pregnancy bedrest with sanity intact can be a challenge for many women and their partners. The goal in this appendix is to provide resources, resources, and more resources! This is a great time to educate yourself about all the things you have wanted to learn, but never seemed to find the time to make happen. The following is a list of resources I hope you find valuable:

BOOKS

Pregnancy:
- *Your Pregnancy Week by Week*, Fifth Edition, by Glade B. Curtis & Judith Schuler
- *What to Expect When You're Expecting*, Third Edition by Heidi Murkoff
- *The Girlfriends' Guide to Pregnancy*, by Vicki Iovine
- *Conception, Pregnancy and Birth*, by Miriam Stoppard
- *Great Expectations*, by Sandy Jones & Marcie Jones
- *Parenting Guide to Pregnancy and Childbirth*, by Paula Spencer
- *Mayo Clinic Complete Book of Pregnancy & Baby's First Year*, by May Clinic
- *Getting Ready for Baby: The Ultimate Organizer for the Mom-To-Be*, by Helene Tragos Stelian
- *The Mother of All Pregnancy Books: The Ultimate Guide to Conception, Birth, and Everything In Between*, by Ann Douglas
- *The Pregnancy Book: Month-by-Month, Everything You Need to Know From America's Baby Experts*, by Martha Sears, et al
- *The Complete Book of Pregnancy and Childbirth (Revised)*, by Sheila Kitzinger

Pregnancy Bedrest:
- *Pregnancy Bedrest: A Guide for the Pregnant Woman and Her Family*, by Susan H. Johnson and Deborah A. Kraut
- *Days In Waiting: A Guide to Surviving Pregnancy Bedrest*, by Mary Ann McCann
- *Bedrest Before Baby: What's a Mother to Do: A Survival Handbook for High Risk Moms*, by Patricia Isennock
- *When Pregnancy Isn't Perfect*, by Laurie A. Rich
- *Preventing Pre-term Birth: A Parent's Guide*, by Michael Katz
- *The High-Risk Pregnancy Sourcebook*, by Denis M. Chism
- *The Pregnancy Bed Rest Book: A Survival Guide for Expectant Mothers and Their Families*, by Amy E. Tracy & Richard H. Schwarz, MD
- *Bedrest Survival Guide*, by Barbara Edelston Peterson
- *Intensive Caring: New Hope for High Risk Pregnancy*, by Dianne Hales & Timothy Johnson, MD
- *Every Pregnant Woman's Guide to Preventing Preterm Birth*, by Barbara Luke
- *And Mommy's On Her Side*, by Heidi Morse-Travis

Multiple Gestation:
- *The Multiple Pregnancy Sourcebook: Pregnancy and the First Days with Twins, Triplets, and More*, by Nancy Bowers
- *Everything You Need To Know To Have A Healthy Twin Pregnancy*, by Gila Leiter, MD
- *When You're Expecting Twins, Triplets, or Quads, Revised Edition: Proven Guidelines for a Healthy Multiple Pregnancy*, by Barbara Luke, Tamara Eberlein, et al
- *Exceptional Pregnancies: A Survival Guide to Parents Expecting Triplets or More*, by Kathleen Birch, et al
- *The Parent's Guide to Raising Twins: From Pre-Birth to First School Days – The Essential Book For All Those Expecting Twins or More*, by Cherry Rowland
- *The Art of Parenting Twins*, by Patricia Maxwell Malmstrom, Janet Poland

Preterm Labor and/or Premature Rupture of Membranes (PROM):
- *Preterm Labor*, by Murdo G., D.Sc., Md. Elder, et al
- *Preterm Birth: Cases, Prevention, and Management*, by Anna-Ritta Fuchs, et

- *The Premature Labor Handbook: Successfully Sustaining Your High-Risk Pregnancy*, by Robertson, Patricia A, MD, et al
- *Getting Pregnant & Staying Pregnant: Overcoming Infertility and Managing Your High-Risk Pregnancy*, by Diana Raab

Gestational Diabetes:
- *Diabetes & Pregnancy: What to Expect*, by Task Force for the American Diabetes Association Council on Pregnancy
- *Gestational Diabetes: What to Expect*, by American Diabetes Association
- *101 Tips for a Healthy Pregnancy with Diabetes*, by Patti Bazel-Geil, et al
- *Medical Management of Pregnancy Complicated by Diabetes (Clinical Education Series)*, by American Diabetes Association
- *Managing Your Gestational Diabetes: A Guide for You and Your Baby's Good Health*, by Lois Jovanovic-Peterson
- *The Official Patient's Sourcebook on Gestational Diabetes*, by James N., MD. & Parker, Philip M., PhD
- *Gestational Diabetes: A Medical Dictionary, Bibliography, and Annotated Research Guide to Internet References*, by Icon Health Publications
- Gestational Diabetes: Guidelines for a Safe Pregnancy and a Healthy baby, by Marion J. Franz

Pre-eclampsia and Eclampsia:
- *Pre-eclampsia: Current Perspective on Management*, by Philip N. Baker, John C.P. Kingdom
- *Pre-Eclampsia: The Facts: The Hidden Threats to Pregnancy (Oxford Medical Publications)*, by Chris Redman, Isabel Walker
- *Pre-Eclampsia: The Hypertensive Disease of Pregnancy*, by Ian Macgillivray

Premature Babies:
- *Preemies: The Essential Guide for Parents of Premature Babies*, by Dana Wechsler Linden
- *Parenting Your Premature Baby and Child: The Emotional Journey*, by Deborah L., PhD, and Mara Tesler Stein
- *Your Premature Baby: The First Five Years*, by Nikki Bradford
- *What To Do When Your Baby Is Premature: A Parent's Handbook for Coping With High-Risk Pregnancy and Caring for the Preterm Infant*, by Joseph A. Garcia-Prats

- *The Premature Baby Book: Everything You Need to Know About Your Premature Baby from Birth to Age One (Sears, William, Sears Parenting Library)*, by James Sears

Nutrition:
- *Pregnancy Nutrition: Good Health for You and Your Baby*, by Elizabeth M. Ward
- *Your Vegetarian Pregnancy: A Month-by Month Guide to Health and Nutrition*, by Holly Roberts
- *Eating Expectantly: Revised and Updated*, by Bridget Swinney
- *The Pregnancy Diet*, by Eileen Behan
- *Fix-it and Forget-it Diabetic Cookbook: Slow Cooker Favorites – To Include Everyone!*, by Phyllis Pellman Good, American Diabetes Association
- *Diabetes Cookbook for Dummies*, by Alan L. Rubin, Fran Stach, Denise C. Sharf
- *Betty Crocker's Diabetes Cookbook: Everyday Meals, Easy as 1-2-3*, by Betty Crocker Editors
- *American Diabetes Association Diabetes Cookbook*, by Sally Mansfield

Breastfeeding:
- *The Breastfeeding Book: Everything You Need to Know About Nursing Your Child From Birth Through Weaning*, by Martha Sears and William Sears
- *The Nursing Mother's Companion*, by Kathleen Huggins
- *So That's What They're For! Breastfeeding Basics*, by Janet Tamaro
- *The Womanly Art of Breastfeeding*, by Gwen Gotsch and Judy Torgus

Babies:
- *What to Expect the First Year*, by Arlene Eisenberg
- *The Baby Book*, by William, Robert, James Sears MD and Martha Sears
- *Your Baby and Child*, by Penelope Leach
- *Taking Care of Baby*, by Caroline Keller and Andrew Lottmann
- *The Portable Pediatrician*, by Laura W. Nathanson
- *Baby Love*, by Robin Barker
- *50 Simple Ways to Pamper Your Baby*, by Karyn Siegel-Maier
- *Baby Matters*, by Linda F. Palmer

Single Mothers:

- *The Complete Single Mother*, by Andrea Engber
- *The Single Mother's Survival Guide*, by Patrice Karst
- *The Single Parent Resource*, by Brook Noel, and Arthur C. Klein
- *Single Mothers by Choice: A Guidebook for Single Women Who are Considering or Have Chosen Motherhood*, by Jane Mattes

Teenage Mothers:

- *Everything You Need to Know About Teen Motherhood*, by Jane Hammerslough
- *Surviving Teen Pregnancy: Your Choices, Dreams, and Decisions*, by Shirley Arthur
- *Coping with Teen Parenting*, by Kay Beyer
- *Teen Pregnancy: The Challenges We Faced, The Choices We Made*, by Donna Ervy

Expectant Fathers:

- *What to Expect When Your Wife is Expecting*, by Thomas Hill and Patrick Merrell
- *The Everything Father-to-Be Book: A Survival Guide for Men (Everything Series)*, by Kevin Nelson
- *The Father's Almanac: From Pregnancy to Pre-School, Baby Care to Behavior, the Complete and Indispensable Book of Practical Advice and Ideas for Every Man Discovering the Fun and Challenge of Fatherhood*, by S. Adams Sullivan
- *Parents Book for New Fathers (Parents Baby Childcare Series)*, by David Laskin
- *The Expectant Father: Facts, Tips and Advice for Dads*, by Armin A. Brott

Self-Help:

- *SOS Help for Emotions: Managing Anxiety, Anger & Depression*, by Lynn Clark, PhD
- *Managing Anxiety*, by Helen Kennerley
- *Anxiety and Depression – A Practical Guide to Recovery*, by Robert Priest
- *Understanding Obsessions and Compulsions*, by Frank Tallis
- *Sibling Bereavement – Helping Children Cope with Loss*, by Ann Farrant
- *The Courage to Grieve – Creative Living, Recovery & Growth Through Grief*, by Judy Tatelbaum

- *Believing in Yourself- A practical Guide to Building Self-Confidence*, by Eric Blumenthal
- *A Woman in Your Own Right: Assertiveness and You*, by Ann Dickson
- *The Dance of Anger*, by Harriet Lerner
- *Mind Over Mood*, by Dennis Greenberger, et al
- *Eating Disorders: Obesity, Anorexia Nervosa, and the Person Within*, by Hilde Bruch
- *Eating Your Heart Out*, by Julia Buckroyd
- *Anorexia Nervosa and the Wish to Change*, by A.H. Crisp, N. Joughin, C. Halek & Bowyer
- *Coping with Bulimia*, by Barbara French
- *Women and Alcohol*, by Elizabeth Ettorre
- *How to Stop Smoking and Stay Stopped for Good*, by Gillian Riley
- *The Road Less Traveled*, by M. Scott Peck
- *Men are From Mars, Women are From Venus*, by John Gray
- *The Dance of Intimacy: A Woman's Guide to Courageous Acts of Change in Key Relationships*, by Harriet Lerner
- *The Good Relationship Guide*, by Dr. Maryon Tysoe
- *The Mirror Within: A New Look at Sexuality*, by Anne Dickson
- *Intimate Partners: Patterns in Love and Marriage*, by Maggie Scarf
- *Meditation*, by Bill Anderton
- *Managing Stress*, by David Fontana
- *The Ultimate Stress Handbook for Women*, by Ursula Markham

MOVIES

Several of these companies have downloadable movies from the internet as well as movie rentals through the mail.

Cinema Now
www.CinemaNow.com

Movieflix
www.Movieflix.com

Movie Link
www.MovieLink.com

Netflix
www.Netflix.com

Wal-Mart DVD Rentals
www.WalMart.com

BlockBuster Online
www.BlockBuster.com

DVD Avenue
www.DVDAvenue.com

Clean Films Edited
www.CleanFilms.com
(popular movies that have been
edited to an "E" rating for family
viewing)

NEWSPAPERS

The following list of websites provides access to news and information
from around the world:

The New York Times Online
www.NewYorkTimes.com

USA Today
www.USAToday.com

Online Newspapers
www.OnlineNewspapers.com

Internet Public Library
www.ipl.org/div/news/

Wall Street Journal
www.WallStreetJournal.com

PRODUCTS FOR BABY & MOTHER

Anne Geddes
www.AnneGeddes.cm

Babinskis
www.Babinskis.com

Baby Bows
www.BabyBows.com

Baby Gap
www.BabyGap.com

Baby Place
www.BabyPlace.com

Wal-Mart
www.WalMart.com

American Baby
www.AmericanBaby.com

Target
www.Target.com

Childrens Place
www.ChildrensPlace.com

Old Navy
www.OldNavy.com

Babies R Us
www.BabiesRUs.com

Gymboree
www.Gymboree.com

Carters
www.Carters.com

Baby Style
www.BabyStyle.com

M3 Preemie Products
www.M3PreemieProducts.com

The Preemie Store
www.Preemie.com

Baby Universe
www.BabyUniverse.com

Baby Safe
www.BabySafe.com

Gap Maternity
www.GapMaternity.com

A Pea in the Pod
www.apeainthepod.com

One Hot Mama
www.onehotmama.com

Mom Shop
www.MomShop.com

Due Maternity
www.DueMaternity.com

Fit Maternity
www.FitMaternity.com

Motherhood Plus
www.motherhoodplus.com

Medela Rental Service
www.Medela.com

Pregnancy Relaxation Essentials
www.PregnancyRelaxationEssentials.com

Pregnancy Bedrest Essentials
www.PregnancyBedrestEssentials.com

PRETERM LABOR AND HIGH RISK PREGNANCY

March of Dimes
Fetal Fibronectin (fFN): A Test for Preterm Delivery
www.marchofdimes.com/professionals/14332_1149.asp

Perinatology.COM
Cervical Incompetence and Cerclage
www.perinatology.com/exposures/maternal/cervix.htm
(this site also has a lot of information about other pregnancy conditions)

American Family Physician
Preterm Labor
www.aafp.org/afp/99020/ap/593.html
(an excellent, comprehensive article)

March of Dimes
Stress and Pregnancy
www.marchofdimes.com/professionals/681_1158.asp

American College of Obstetrics and Gynecologists
www.acog.com

Medline Plus
High Risk Pregnancy
www.nlm.nih.gov/medlineplus/highriskpregnancy.htm/

Medline Plus
Diabetes and Pregnancy
www.nlm.nih.gov/medlineplus/diabetesandpregnancy.htm/

American Diabetes Association
Gestational Diabetes
www.diabetes.org/home.jsp

Pre-eclampsia Foundation
www.preeclampsia.org

Medline Plus
High Blood Pressure in Pregnancy
www.nlm.nih.gov/medlineplus/highbloodpressureinpregnancy.html

HER Foundation
Hyperemesis Gravidarum
www.helpher.org

American Pregnancy Association
Placenta Previa
www.americanpregnancy.org/pregnancycomplications/placentaprevia.html

March of Dimes
Placental Abruption
www.marchofdimes.com/pnhec/188_1135.asp

American Family Physician
Intrauterine Growth Retardation (IUGR)
www.aafp.org/afp/981015ap/vandenbo.html

Emedicine
Premature Rupture of Membranes (PROM)
www.emedicine.com/med/topic3246.htm

MULTIPLE GESTATION

March of Dimes
Multiples: Twins, Triplets and Beyond
www.marchofdimes.com/professionals/681_4545.asp

The Triplet Connection
Management of Multiple Gestations
www.tripletconnection.org/gestations.html

Marvelous Multiples
www.MarvelousMultiples.com

PREGNANCY BEDREST

Pregnancy Bedrest Essentials
www.PregnancyBedrestEssentials.com

Sidelines
www.sidelines.org

Surviving Pregnancy Bedrest
www.childbirthsolutions.com/articles/pregnancy/bedrest/indes.php

Moms on Bedrest
www.momsonbedrest.com

Baby Zone
www.BabyZone.com

CHILDBIRTHING TECHNIQUES

Lamaze International
www.lamaze-childbirth.com

The Alexander Technique
www.AlexanderTechnique.com

The Bradley Method
www.bradleybirth.com

Hypnosis
www.hypnobirthing.com

Video Childbirth Class
www.ChildbirthClass.com

Lamaze Video
www.MaternityMarketing.com

BABY NAMES

Baby Name Meanings
www.baby-names-meanings.com

A-Z Baby Names
www.a-zbabynames.com

All Girl Baby Names
www.allgirlbabynames.com

All Boy Baby Names
www.allboybabynames.com

Alternative Baby Names
www.alternativebabynames.com

BREAST FEEDING

La Leche League
www.lalecheleague.org

4 Women.Gov
www.4women.gov/breastfeeding/index.htm

American Baby
www.americanbaby.com/home/breastfeeding.html

PREGNANCY LOSS

Mommies Enduring Neonatal Death
www.mend.org

Hannah's Prayer Ministries
www.hannah.org

Share: Pregnancy and Infant Loss Support
www.nationalshareoffice.com

Born Angels: Pregnancy Loss Support
www.bornangels.com

Fertility Plus: Miscarriage Support
www.fertilityplus.org

Multiples Angels Network
www.angels4ever.com

DOMESTIC VIOLENCE

The National Domestic Violence Hotline
1-800-779-7233
www.ndvh.org

Crisis Support Network
http://crisis-support.org

Domestic Violence Notepad (excellent list of resources)
www.womenlaw.com/domestic.htm

PUBLIC ASSISTANCE FOR MONEY AND FOOD

Welfare Information Network
www.financeprojectinfo.org.win

Food & Nutrition Service (Food Stamp Program)
www.fns.usda.gov/fsp/

Women, Infants and Children (WIC)
www.fns.usda.gov/wic/

Appendix B

Baby's Activity Record

⋖⋗⋖⋗⋖⋗⋖⋗⋖⋗⋖⋗⋖⋗

Around the 7th month of pregnancy (28 weeks gestation), OB/GYNs encourage the expectant mother to begin monitoring her baby's movements; this process is better known as kick counting. It is important for the expectant mother to get to know her baby's movements so she knows how her baby is developing and can report any changes in activity to her doctor. Healthy babies tend to be active throughout the day, sleeping for short periods of time. Each baby has its own special time of day it will be most active, maybe after breakfast or lunch, after the mother showers, or upon the mother's awaking. Activity is usually noted in the form of kicks, rolls, twists, and turns. For the most part, a healthy baby usually moves at least 10 times in a two (2) hour period.

Various ways exist to monitor a baby's movements in utero, and most OB/GYNs have a particular preference for monitoring baby's movements in their patients. Talk with your doctor and ask which method he or she prefers and implement it into your daily routine. Your baby's activity should be monitored around the same time each day.

I have provided, in this section, weekly kick count charts from twenty-eight (28) weeks gestation to forty (40) weeks gestation. These weekly charts are based on the concept of 10 movements within a two hour time frame. Again, you will want to speak with your doctor to determine which method of baby activity monitoring is preferred. Also, keep in mind that some medications prescribed for medically challenged pregnancies can affect the baby's activity. Talk with your OB/GYN about your specific medications and what you can expect in relation to side effects of medications on your baby.

Also remember to call your doctor if you have any concerns about your baby's activity level. He or she will be able to address your concerns and to relieve your anxiety.

Counting Your Baby's Movements

- Choose a time when your baby is usually active. Most babies tend to become active after meals, so this might be the best time to monitor your baby's activity level. Keep in mind, you will want to monitor around the same time each day.
- Reduce as much noise as possible in your living space.
- Position yourself on the left side with your hands placed on your abdomen.
- Write down the date and time you begin monitoring your baby's activity.
- Continue counting until the baby has moved 10 times. Count all movements: kicks, rolls, twists, and turns.
- After counting 10 movements, write down the stop time on the chart and exactly how many minutes it took to feel 10 movements.

If your baby has not moved 10 times within two hours, or you notice a significant decrease in your baby's activity, call your doctor right away. The following charts will help you monitor your baby's activity and hopefully provide peace of mind as well.

27 Weeks Gestation							
Day	Sun	Mon	Tue	Wed	Thu	Fri	Sat
Date	5/1/05	5/2/05	5/3/05	5/4/05	5/5/05	5/6/05	5/7/05
Start Time	8:00am	8:00am	8:00am	8:00am	8:00am	8:00am	8:00am
Stop Time	8:42am	8:35am	8:58am	9:10am	8:45am	9:00am	8:52am
10 Kicks	42min	35min	58min	70min	45 min	60min	52min

28 Weeks Gestation							
Day	Sun	Mon	Tue	Wed	Thu	Fri	Sat
Date							
Start Time							
Stop Time							
10 Kicks							

29 Weeks Gestation							
Day	Sun	Mon	Tue	Wed	Thu	Fri	Sat
Date							
Start Time							
Stop Time							
10 Kicks							

30 Weeks Gestation

Day	Sun	Mon	Tue	Wed	Thu	Fri	Sat
Date							
Start Time							
Stop Time							
10 Kicks							

31 Weeks Gestation

Day	Sun	Mon	Tue	Wed	Thu	Fri	Sat
Date							
Start Time							
Stop Time							
10 Kicks							

32 Weeks Gestation

Day	Sun	Mon	Tue	Wed	Thu	Fri	Sat
Date							
Start Time							
Stop Time							
10 Kicks							

33 Weeks Gestation

Day	Sun	Mon	Tue	Wed	Thu	Fri	Sat
Date							
Start Time							
Stop Time							
10 Kicks							

34 Weeks Gestation

Day	Sun	Mon	Tue	Wed	Thu	Fri	Sat
Date							
Start Time							
Stop Time							
10 Kicks							

35 Weeks Gestation

Day	Sun	Mon	Tue	Wed	Thu	Fri	Sat
Date							
Start Time							
Stop Time							
10 Kicks							

36 Weeks Gestation

Day	Sun	Mon	Tue	Wed	Thu	Fri	Sat
Date							
Start Time							
Stop Time							
10 Kicks							

37 Weeks Gestation

Day	Sun	Mon	Tue	Wed	Thu	Fri	Sat
Date							
Start Time							
Stop Time							
10 Kicks							

38 Weeks Gestation

Day	Sun	Mon	Tue	Wed	Thu	Fri	Sat
Date							
Start Time							
Stop Time							
10 Kicks							

39 Weeks Gestation

Day	Sun	Mon	Tue	Wed	Thu	Fri	Sat
Date							
Start Time							
Stop Time							
10 Kicks							

40 Weeks Gestation

Day	Sun	Mon	Tue	Wed	Thu	Fri	Sat
Date							
Start Time							
Stop Time							
10 Kicks							

Notes

Notes